50 things you today to manage
eczema

Wendy Green

Foreword by Helen Pugsley,
Dermatology Lecturer, Cardiff University

PERSONAL HEALTH GUIDES

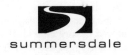

summersdale

50 THINGS YOU CAN DO TODAY TO MANAGE ECZEMA

Summersdale Publishers Ltd
46 West Street
Chichester
West Sussex
PO19 1RP
UK

www.summersdale.com

Printed and bound in Great Britain

ISBN: 978-1-84024-721-3

Disclaimer
Every effort has been made to ensure that the information in this book is accurate and current at the time of publication. The author and the publisher cannot accept responsibility for any misuse or misunderstanding of any information contained herein, or any loss, damage or injury, be it health, financial or otherwise, suffered by any individual or group acting upon or relying on information contained herein. None of the opinions or suggestions in this book is intended to replace medical opinion. If you have concerns about your health, please seek professional advice.

To my husband Gordon, for being so supportive

Acknowledgements

I'd like to thank Helen Pugsley, dermatology lecturer at Cardiff University, for her expert advice – particularly regarding medications for the treatment of eczema. I'm also grateful to Jennifer Barclay for being understanding and easy to work with and to Laura Booth for helping me to organise the information.

Contents

Author's Note..9

Foreword by Helen Pugsley, Dermatology Lecturer...........11

Introduction...13

Chapter 1 – Eczema Explained...15

1. Identify your eczema triggers

Chapter 2 – Skin Deep...31

2. Keep your skin moist with emollients

3. Try other medications

4. Try alternative treatments

5. Prepare for the sun

6. Take care of your skin in the water

7. Dress sensibly

8. Identify when you scratch

9. Stop scratching

Chapter 3 – Inside Out..56

10. Keep your skin well hydrated
11. Nourish your skin with a balanced diet
12. Supplement your diet
13. Identify your food allergies
14. Be aware of food additives
15. Eat the right foods during pregnancy and childhood
16. Learn from others' experiences with food
17. Keep a food diary
18. Take a skin test
19. Sleep well with the right bedtime foods and drink

Chapter 4 – Eczema and Emotions.......................................80

20. Identify your stress triggers
21. Just say no
22. Be assertive
23. Accept what you can't change
24. Change your perception
25. Manage your time
26. Eat a de-stress diet
27. Get moving
28. Get back to nature
29. Laugh more
30. Breathe deep
31. Focus on the here and now
32. Meditate

33. Find social support
34. Sleep well

Chapter 5 – Home Front...**97**

35. Control dust mites
36. Control temperature
37. Solve your pet problems
38. Glove up
39. Clean naturally
40. Use non-biological washing powders
41. Use water softeners

Chapter 6 – DIY Complementary Therapies......................**107**

42. Use essential oils
43. Help yourself with homeopathy
44. Try hypnotherapy
45. Visualise healthy skin
46. Enjoy a massage
47. Turn to naturopathy
48. Try flower remedies
49. Find relief in reflexology
50. Say 'yes' to yoga

Jargon Buster...**120**
Useful Products..**123**
Helpful Books...**133**
Directory...**135**

Author's Note

I've suffered from atopic eczema and contact irritant dermatitis since my early twenties. Prior to that I'd had hay fever – when that disappeared, the eczema seemed to replace it. The atopic eczema mainly affects my face and neck – including the insides of my ears and my eyelids, which become swollen, as well as extremely itchy and sore. Over the years I've realised that stress is my main trigger. A few years ago, during a prolonged stressful period at work, I had a particularly bad flare-up that barely responded to the hydrocortisone cream my GP prescribed.

I've since found that the best way for me to minimise flare-ups is to keep a handle on stress. I've also benefited from supplements, having experienced fewer flare-ups since taking evening primrose oil and fish oil capsules daily. Washing with aqueous cream and wearing rubber gloves for the household chores seems to reduce episodes of irritant contact dermatitis.

Eczema is an individual condition – what works for one person may not work for another. In this book I've suggested a variety of both conventional and alternative treatments and techniques that can help you to control your eczema. You may need to try a few before you find the right combination.

Wendy Green

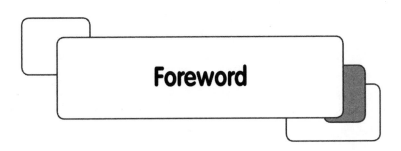

Foreword

by Helen Pugsley, dermatology lecturer, Cardiff University

It is thought that one in seven people will suffer from some kind of eczema in their lifetime. Skin has such an important function – it's not there just to hold in our vital organs. Many underestimate the social function that skin has and the first impressions we may have of someone who has a chronic skin disease like eczema.

This book provides a superb overview of eczema and in particular offers helpful hints to a healthy lifestyle, which ultimately helps patients and carers to cope with the condition.

The layout is simple to follow and it is easy to see where the author has used clinical evidence, anecdotal evidence, patients' experiences and case studies from experts that are nicely summarised to provide useful information that is easily understood.

The book covers a few key areas that have caused controversy and debate amongst experts for many years, but the author has managed to present an unbiased and sensible approach that does not promise the unachievable or suggest a miraculous cure.

The advice is up to date with current clinical research and the author has presented a holistic approach that is entirely appropriate for a self-help guide, offering the reader all they need to know to combine conventional and complementary treatments with a healthy lifestyle.

Introduction

Evidence suggests that in the past 30 years or so the number of eczema sufferers has more than doubled – one in five children and one in 12 adults in the UK now suffer from some form of the condition. Some experts believe this increase may be due to aspects of modern lifestyles such as central heating and exposure to chemicals in toiletries, cosmetics and household cleaners, as well as pollution and food additives.

Famous eczema sufferers include Ulrika Jonsson, who said recently that she suffered from eczema as a child and used to rub her eyelids until they became so swollen she couldn't see, and that she still has scars in the creases of her knees and arms. The actress Claire Sweeney has revealed that she gets eczema on her face. Other well-known sufferers include Brad Pitt, Nadia Sawalha, LeAnn Rimes and Jade Jagger.

This book explains how psychological, dietary, hormonal and environmental factors can play a part in eczema and offers practical advice and a holistic approach to help you deal with your symptoms. You'll discover how simple lifestyle and dietary changes can help to prevent and treat flare-ups. You'll learn how best to care for your skin and adapt your home environment. Simple stress management strategies and techniques from complementary therapies are also included. At the end of the book you'll find details of helpful products, books and organisations.

Chapter 1

Eczema Explained

This chapter gives you an overview of the types, sites, symptoms and possible causes of eczema, along with advice to help you identify your triggers. Specific advice on each of these triggers is provided in the relevant chapters.

What is eczema?

Eczema is the name given to a group of conditions where the skin is irritated or inflamed. Also known as dermatitis – which literally means skin inflammation – it is an uncomfortable, often distressing complaint. It can affect the whole body, or just certain areas. Common sites include the backs of the hands and knees, behind the ears and the fronts of the elbows and hands. Although eczema can resemble some infectious skin conditions, it is not contagious.

Identifying eczema

Your eczema symptoms will obviously depend on the type you are suffering from, but these are the common signs.

Skin inflammation – a characteristic of all types of eczema. Skin becomes red, sore and swollen.

Itching – if your skin doesn't itch, you probably don't have eczema. Itching tends to lead to scratching, which can make the inflammation worse and lead to the skin splitting and becoming infected. Once infected, the skin may crack and weep, a condition known as 'wet' eczema.

Dry and scaly skin – can be both a cause and an effect of eczema.

Blisters – also known as vesicles. These occur mainly on the hands and feet and are caused by an allergic reaction, which results in fluid building up in the skin tissues. The blisters can burst and weep and become crusty.

Thickened skin – chronic scratching and rubbing can lead to the skin producing more of a protein called keratin in an attempt to protect itself. This eventually leads to lichenification – where the skin becomes thickened, leathery and scaly, with exaggerated creases.

Impetigo – can be a complication of eczema, because it often results from broken skin. It is a bacterial skin infection that develops when staphylococcus bacteria, normally present on the skin's surface or, more rarely, streptococcus bacteria, enter broken skin and multiply, causing blistering and crusting. Small blisters develop first, which tend to burst, leaving moist, yellow crusts. Impetigo patches are usually small and itchy. The infection can spread quickly because scratching leads to the bacteria being transferred to other parts of the body via the fingernails. Impetigo is spread through contact, so any affected individuals should use their own towels and facecloths.

Note:

If you suspect that you or a child has impetigo, you should see your GP as soon as possible, who will usually prescribe either a bactericidal ointment or an oral antibiotic.

Types of eczema

There are various types of eczema, the two most common being atopic eczema and irritant contact dermatitis. Other forms of the condition include allergic contact dermatitis, discoid eczema, seborrhoeic eczema, dyshydrotic dermatitis, gravitational (varicose) eczema and photosensitive (light sensitive) eczema.

Atopic eczema

Atopic, or allergic eczema, is the most common type and is thought to be inherited. If one or both of your parents, or a brother, sister or grandparent are atopic – i.e. suffer from eczema, asthma or hay fever – you have an increased risk of suffering from atopic eczema. In atopy, an overreaction by the immune system leads to inflamed, irritated and sore skin.

Atopic eczema is commonest in childhood, especially during the first five years of life. It tends to improve with age; however, some people still continue to suffer from it in adulthood. It's thought that people with atopic eczema are sensitive to allergens in the environment which others find harmless. Allergens include pet dander (skin flakes), house dust mite droppings, moulds and pollens (see Chapter 5) and foods such as eggs, shellfish and soya (see Chapter 3). Stress is also thought to exacerbate symptoms (see Chapter 4). A common feature is itching, which can be extreme. Other symptoms include dryness, redness and inflammation and there can be blisters which burst and leak fluid. Scratching can cause the skin to split and leave it open to infection. Atopic eczema can occur almost anywhere on the body, but it most often affects the head, face, neck, arms, backs of knees and the toes...

Irritant contact dermatitis
This type of eczema is caused by regular contact with everyday substances, like soap, detergents and chemicals, which damage the skin by removing the oils, fats and proteins that normally form a protective barrier. Once this happens moisture is lost from the skin, leaving it dry, itchy and irritated. This leaves the deeper layers of skin exposed to substances, which cause further irritation, cracking and chapping. Common irritants include water – especially hard water, soap, washing up liquids, foam baths and shower creams and household cleaners such as bleach. Others include caustic soda, paint stripper, white spirit and gardening chemicals. It occurs most often on adults' hands and is best prevented by avoiding irritants and keeping the skin well moisturised. Avoiding irritating substances can be difficult because we use our hands to do so many things in day-to-day life. Unfortunately, lots of professions also involve having to wash your hands often, or using chemicals, for example nursing and hairdressing. It can be especially difficult when it does occur in children, as they tend to be exposed to potential irritants such as paints, sand and play dough whilst at nursery and school. Hand eczema can also be embarrassing, because the hands are usually on display. For more helpful advice see Chapter 5 – Home Front. For tips on skin care see Chapter 2 – Skin Deep.

Allergic contact dermatitis

This form of eczema develops when the body's immune system overreacts to a substance that comes in contact with the skin. The allergic reaction may develop over a period of time after repeated contact with the substance. For example, about five per cent of people have an allergic reaction to nickel, often found in earrings, belt buckles and the buttons on jeans. Reactions may occur after contact with other substances like perfumes, make-up, rubber, sticking plasters, glues, dyes, resins and plants. The eczema occurs anywhere on the body that is exposed to the offending substance.

If you suspect your eczema is due to contact with a particular substance, you can ask your GP to refer you to a dermatology clinic for a patch test. This test involves applying the suspected allergens to the skin using circular test patches. These are left on for two days. On removal, any reactions – such as reddening, a rash or blistering – are noted and interpreted.

Discoid eczema

This type of eczema mainly occurs in adults and can appear suddenly as a few coin shaped areas of red, intensely itchy skin, normally on the trunk or limbs. These areas can weep fluid and may become infected. Preventative action might involve avoiding irritating substances and using emollients. However, during a flare-up, a strong hydrocortisone cream is usually needed. Often a preparation that also contains an antibiotic is necessary, as this type of eczema is more likely to harbour bacterial infections. Combined creams include Betnovate C and Fucidin H, both of which are only available on prescription.

Seborrhoeic eczema

This type of eczema tends to affect people between the ages of 15 and 45. It usually appears on the scalp as mild dandruff, but may spread to the face, especially oily areas at the sides of the nose and on the eyebrows, ears, including the ear canal, and chest. The skin becomes red and inflamed and begins to flake. The condition is thought to be due to an overgrowth of yeast on the skin. It may also be hormone-related, as it often flares up in premenstrual women. Exposure to sunlight can help to reduce symptoms, though in some people it can trigger photosensitive (light-sensitive) eczema. There's no clinical evidence that excluding certain foods is of any benefit. Other self-help treatments include an anti-fungal cream, such as clotrimazole or mild hydrocortisone cream, both of which are available over the counter in pharmacies. Your GP may prescribe a scalp ointment, or a tar-based shampoo.

Infantile seborrhoeic eczema
Otherwise known as cradle cap, this is a common condition in babies under one year old. Characterised by greasy, yellow scales, it usually starts on the scalp or in the nappy area and spreads quickly. Despite looking unpleasant, this type of eczema isn't sore or itchy and doesn't cause discomfort. It usually clears up in a few months, but can continue for several years. Emollients or olive oil may help to remove the scales. If it becomes infected, see your GP.

Dyshydrotic dermatitis
Dyshydrotic dermatitis, otherwise known as pompholyx, is a type of hand eczema that occurs twice as often in women as men. It starts as intense itching or burning on the hands or feet, or both, and then tiny blisters erupt along the sides of the fingers and may also appear on the palms and soles. It's thought there may be a link with abnormal sweating in the affected areas. The rash can last for up to four weeks. Steroid cream usually helps to control the itching. Scratching the blisters can lead to them bursting and oozing fluid, and exposing raw skin beneath. Antibiotics may be needed if the

affected areas become infected. It may be triggered by stress, contact with irritants, such as household cleaners, or an allergy to drugs, such as neomycin, or to nickel.

Gravitational (varicose) eczema

Gravitational eczema affects the lower legs of middle-aged and older people. It's caused by poor circulation. The skin around the ankles is usually affected, becoming itchy, red and scaly. The eczema needs to be treated or the skin may break down, leading to an ulcer. As is the case with most forms of eczema, the usual treatment is with emollients and steroid creams. Wearing compression stockings and avoiding standing for long periods may help prevent further flare-ups.

Photosensitive (light sensitive) eczema

Photosensitive eczema is triggered when the skin is exposed to the sun. Because the face is usually uncovered it tends to be particularly vulnerable. The resulting rash can be itchy and red and is sometimes sore and weepy. This form of eczema is sometimes triggered by the use of certain medications, such as antihistamines, and chemicals which interact with the sun's rays. Your GP may suggest alternative medications, the use of a sunblock or refer you to a dermatologist.

Eczema sites

Facial eczema

Of all the sites where eczema can erupt, the face is probably the most visible and therefore facial eczema is likely to be the most embarrassing form of the condition. It can be one of several types of eczema – atopic, seborrhoeic, or irritant and allergic contact dermatitis. Atopic eczema is the commonest cause of facial eczema. It often appears on the cheeks and forehead first, but the whole face, including the upper and lower eyelids, can be involved. The eyelids can become swollen and the skin thickened, with the normal creases appearing more pronounced.

Seborrhoeic eczema can often affect the sides of the nose, inner eyebrows and sometimes the eyelids.

Irritant contact eczema on the face may be caused by anything that dries out the skin's protective barrier, including soap, overly harsh skin cleansers and toners, hard water and men's products like shaving foam and aftershave. The solution is to use unperfumed, hypoallergenic skincare products – well-known brands include Simple, Almay and Clinique. Alternatively, you could use emulsifying ointment, or aqueous cream instead of soap and as a substitute for shaving foam, or shaving soap. Men might also benefit from using an alcohol-free aftershave balm – most men's grooming ranges include them.

Allergic contact dermatitis on the face may be caused by direct contact with a sensitising chemical found in cosmetics – make-up, skin care products and hair dyes – and contact with airborne substances such as perfume sprays and pollen. Nickel allergy can causes eczema on the ear lobes and occasionally metal spectacle frames can be to blame. Perfume oils, which are free of alcohol, may be less drying and irritating than conventional alcohol-based fragrances. The Body Shop offers a range of perfume oils.

Cosmetics often contain sensitisers (substances that can provoke an allergic reaction), such as lanolin, fragrance, dyes and preservatives. Many women will find that their skin can tolerate hypoallergenic make-up by companies like Almay and Clinique. Mineral make-up, made from crushed minerals such as on titanium dioxide and zinc oxide, is said to be less irritating to sensitive skin than conventional make-up. They're also claimed to present virtually no allergy risk and to have a soothing, calming, anti-inflammatory effect on the skin, making them ideal if you suffer from facial eczema. Titanium dioxide is a natural sunscreen, whilst zinc oxide helps to heal the skin. Iredale Mineral Cosmetics and Lily Lolo Mineral Cosmetics offer a wide range of mineral make-up products. For further details see the Useful Products section. Mineral make-up is also available from high street make-up brands like Maybelline and Max Factor.

Scalp eczema

Eczema on the scalp can be caused by the atopic, seborrhoeic and irritant contact forms. Your GP may recommend a pomade, or a coal tar shampoo. If you suspect it is caused by contact with an irritant, consider changing to a mild shampoo and conditioner. Most proprietary dry skin ranges include scalp shampoos and treatments. Hair dye is another possible irritant to consider. See the Useful Products section for more information.

What else could it be?

There are other skin conditions that you could possibly mistake for eczema. Some of these are outlined below. If you're at all in doubt about the cause of your rash, visit your GP, who will be able to make an accurate diagnosis.

Ichthyosis

Ichthyosis is a rare condition that involves the continual and widespread scaling of the skin. It can be genetic, or it can develop at any age, usually as a result of another medical problem, such as kidney disease. In the commonest form – ichthyosis vulgaris – the skin is dry and thickened, with fine white scales. The main difference between ichthyosis and eczema is that the scaling affects most areas of the skin and remains roughly the same over the years, whereas in eczema only certain areas are affected and it tends to change its pattern quite often.

Psoriasis

In psoriasis the rash is less itchy than that of eczema and the thickened red or pink dry patches are more clearly defined, with silvery scales. The rash tends to appear on the elbows and knees, but sometimes the shins, lower back and scalp can be affected.

Rashes with fever

These are common in childhood and often connected with illnesses such as German measles or meningitis. The most obvious difference is that they're linked to other symptoms, such as fever. In German measles there are also flu-like symptoms. The rash consists of many tiny, raised spots that merge together. The rash of meningococcal meningitis appears as purple patches that don't fade when a glass is pressed against them and it isn't itchy. Always seek medical help immediately if you suspect meningitis.

Ringworm

Ringworm (tinea) is a fungal infection characterised by ring or oval-shaped scaly, itchy patches, which could be mistaken for eczema. However, the rash differs in that the 'ring' has a red edge and the skin inside it looks normal, perhaps with only a little scaling. The commonest form is athlete's foot, but other types can appear elsewhere on the body.

The infection is spread by personal contact. People who come into close contact with animals are also at risk. Your GP may take a skin scraping to make a diagnosis. Ringworm is usually treated with antifungal cream or tablets.

Scabies

Scabies is a mite infestation under the upper layer of skin that causes an extremely itchy, lumpy, red rash. The itch and rash are caused by a reaction to the mites. Common sites for infestation include the palms and soles, between the fingers and toes, the skin around the navel, the wrists and the armpits. Scabies may trigger eczema. Treatment is with 5 per cent Permethrin cream or a malathion liquid such as Derbac-M – both of which can be bought over the counter at pharmacies.

It is sometimes difficult to tell the difference between a rash caused by scabies and other skin conditions, such as eczema. Your GP may take a scraping from the skin and send it to the lab if there is any doubt about the diagnosis.

Urticaria

Urticaria is caused by the release of histamine in the skin and is characterised by red or pink weals that look similar to nettle stings. The weals are itchy and may be surrounded by red or pink raised areas. The skin isn't usually dry and scaly, as in eczema, and doesn't ooze, unless scratching leads to the skin breaking.

The three stages of eczema

An additional way of classifying eczema is to describe the stage it's at.

Acute – is when the eczema has just flared up and is likely to be red, possibly with blisters and some oozing or crusts.

Chronic – is when the skin has been eczematous for a while and is likely to be thickened, dry, scaly and cracked.

Infected – is when bacteria has entered broken skin and can happen at the acute or chronic stage.

Causes of eczema

All in the genes?

Research suggests that a genetic mutation that switches off the filaggrin gene leads to dry, scaly skin and predisposes some people to atopic eczema. Filaggrin is a protein which helps to form a barrier on the skin's surface to keep water in, and foreign substances out. A reduction or absence of filaggrin has a detrimental effect on the formation of the skin barrier, leading to the skin drying out too easily and flaking off, allowing foreign substances to enter the skin and cause inflammation. It is thought around five million people in the UK have a filaggrin mutation and as a result have dry skin, which predisposes them to eczema.

What is atopy?

Atopy means allergy and, like the filaggrin gene mutation, is thought to be inherited. A person who is atopic has, in effect, an oversensitive immune system which wrongly identifies substances like pollen or pet dander as a threat to the body and then overreacts by producing too much of an antibody called Immunoglobulin E – IgE for short. Antibodies are proteins circulating in the bloodstream that are involved in the immune response. IgE binds to offending substances to allow other antibodies to remove them. This ignites a chain of chemical reactions in the body, known as inflammation. If you're predisposed to eczema, the inflammation manifests itself in the skin as swelling, redness and itching.

The sensitisation process

An allergic reaction doesn't normally happen the first time you encounter an allergen. Your body has to 'learn' how to react, or become sensitised, to the allergen over a period of time.

First of all, your body comes into contact with an allergen, which the blood cells involved in your immune response perceive as a threat. Over the days or weeks that follow, your body produces allergic antibodies, which attach themselves to mast cells in your body's tissues. Mast cells produce a chemical called histamine, which is designed to aid the removal of the offending agents and leads to inflammation and the associated itching, redness and swelling. The next time your body encounters the allergen, your immune system immediately 'recognises' it as an enemy and leaps into action, resulting in allergic symptoms, such as eczema.

Other factors

Whilst it seems that you can inherit a predisposition to suffer from eczema, dietary, psychological, hormonal and environmental factors may also be involved in bringing on symptoms. Although there's little you can do about genetic predisposition, you can adopt lifestyle changes that could help to minimise attacks.

Some sufferers claim they have improved their symptoms by either changing their diet or by supplementing it. There's some evidence that psychological factors also play a part – many sufferers and health professionals believe there's a link between stress and flare-ups. Some experts believe that how we deal with our emotions can also be a factor in eczema. Eczema in women can sometimes worsen as a result of hormonal changes linked to menstruation. Many believe that our environment can play a part, citing the chemicals in our homes as a major factor in the increasing number of eczema sufferers. Contact with allergens such as pollen or house dust mites can trigger a flare-up in some people.

1. Identify your eczema triggers

Knowing what your triggers are is fundamental to finding ways of managing your eczema. Some experts believe that each sufferer has a threshold to which various factors contribute, and that when there are enough of these contributory factors present at one time an eczema flare-up is likely. For example, your main triggers may be pollen and stress. Pollen alone may not be enough to trigger an attack, but if you are suffering a stressful event at a time when pollen levels are high, the two factors combined may be enough to spark an attack.

If you haven't already identified your triggers, try keeping a trigger diary – a small notebook that you can carry around with you will do the job. Record any potential triggers in it and any eczema symptoms. Eventually, you should be able to link specific factors to your eczema flare-ups.

Common Triggers

Eczema is an individual condition. Various triggers have been identified. These include:

Allergens

Pollen, house dust mite droppings, feathers or fur and pets' dander (skin scales)

Certain foods and medications

Irritants

- Fabrics like wool or synthetics

- Soap, cosmetics and perfumes

- Detergents, household cleaners and air fresheners

- Cigarette smoke and dust

Other triggers

- Hard water, central heating, extreme heat (e.g. hot baths) or extreme cold

- Excessive sweating, a damp or dry atmosphere

- Swimming baths (chlorinated water)

- Stress, tiredness, suppressed emotions

- Poor diet

- Menstruation

- Pregnancy

- Menopause

- Illness and skin infections

Note: It's thought that around half of pregnant women who suffered with eczema before becoming pregnant will find their symptoms worsen and about a quarter will find they improve. Naturally, pregnancy will affect the type of treatment your GP will recommend – emollients, weak hydrocortisone creams and ultraviolet B therapy are deemed safe, but other treatments such as oral steroids should be used with caution and some other medications, including ultraviolet A therapy, are viewed as unsafe.

A holistic approach

This book presents lots of tips and techniques which may help you to reduce and treat your symptoms – some are scientifically proven, whilst others are supported by anecdotal evidence only. The underlying philosophy is that the best way to reduce eczema flare-ups is to take a holistic approach. This might include caring for your skin by keeping it clean and moisturised, using scratch-reduction techniques, avoiding exposure to irritants and allergens, adapting your diet, managing your stress levels and dealing with your emotions effectively. The secret is to find out what works best for you and your particular symptoms.

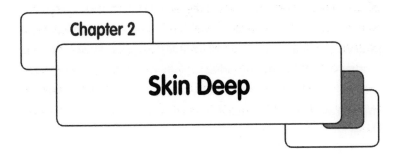

Skin Deep

This chapter looks at what skin is, what it does and how it functions. It will examine how best to care for your skin to prevent flare-ups and to alleviate the dryness and itching that accompanies eczema. There is also an overview of the different medications your GP might prescribe to either prevent or treat your eczema symptoms.

Skin: What it is

Your skin is an amazing organ that weighs around three to five kilograms and if spread out would cover an area of roughly two square metres. Each square metre of your skin has around 200 sensory receptors, 15 sebaceous glands, 100 sweat glands, 70 centimetres of blood vessels and 55 centimetres of nerves. It's strong yet flexible, waterproof yet absorbent, resilient, washable and self-repairing.

Your skin is made up of an outer layer, the epidermis, and an inner layer of fibrous tissue called the dermis. Under the dermis is subcutaneous tissue, in which fat is stored for energy and insulation. Tough and waterproof, the epidermis is made up of layers of dead skin cells, which are constantly being sloughed off and replaced with new ones moving up from the dermis. Its purpose is to protect the more delicate living cells of the dermis below. The dermis contains blood vessels, nerves, sweat glands and muscle tissue and supports and nourishes the epidermis.

Throughout your skin's layers are cells that form part of your immune system; some detect foreign proteins, such as bacteria or viruses, whilst others destroy and remove them. Certain cells produce proteins called antibodies, which in effect trap the foreign proteins – other cells then move in and destroy them. As already mentioned, in people who suffer from atopic eczema, this immune response is hypersensitive and as a result overreacts to substances perceived as a threat.

Skin: What it does

Skin provides a protective barrier between you and the surrounding environment, preventing water and other bodily fluids from being lost and keeping infections out. The natural oils (sebum) in your skin contribute by preventing moisture from evaporating and curbing the growth of bacteria. Your skin's other functions include detecting and regulating your temperature, enabling you to sense, touch and feel the world around you, excreting your body's waste through sweat, producing vitamin D and signalling emotions such as embarrassment, shock and fear.

With eczema, the skin's protective barrier is weakened and the skin becomes irritated and inflamed.

Visiting your GP

For many people, eating a healthy diet, managing stress, dealing with emotions, getting adequate sleep and avoiding irritants and allergens will be enough to reduce the number and severity of eczema flare-ups. However, there are still likely to be occasions when you need to visit your GP. Situations that are likely to require medical diagnosis, treatment and advice include when you have – or suspect you have –

eczema for the first time, when it fails to respond to lifestyle changes and over-the-counter treatments, or if it becomes infected. As well as emollients, there's quite a wide range of medications available for the treatment of eczema. Some, such as hydrocortisone and aqueous creams, are available over the counter, whilst others, such as oral steroids, are only available on prescription.

When you visit your GP it's probably a good idea to take any records you have of your eczema attacks – e.g. how often they happen, how long they last, what triggers, if any, you've identified, which over-the-counter remedies you've tried, etc.

2. Keep your skin moist with emollients

One of the best ways to prevent eczema flare-ups is to keep your skin soft and supple by applying an emollient every day. Emollients are oil or fat based and can come in the form of a cream, ointment, lotion or bath and shower oil. They don't hydrate the skin, as is commonly thought. They work by acting as a barrier that reduces the amount of moisture your skin loses. For this reason they are best used to prevent dry skin rather than to treat it. This means they are most effective when applied frequently, even when your skin is healthy, to minimise flare-ups. The British Association of Dermatologists (BAD) recommends the application of emollients every four hours or at least three to four times daily. Some emollients have anti-inflammatory and anti-itching benefits as well.

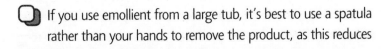 If you use emollient from a large tub, it's best to use a spatula rather than your hands to remove the product, as this reduces

the risk of introducing bacteria, which could cause skin infections. Ensuring that you wash your hands before applying the product also reduces the risk of infection.

Get in the habit of applying an emollient immediately after washing, showering or bathing, to keep moisture in. Apply it last thing at night to improve the condition of problem areas.

Store your emollient in the fridge if your skin is especially hot and itchy. It makes it even more cooling and soothing.

If the product you use comes in a large tub, put some in a small pot or jar. Empty face or hand cream pots, miniature jam jars or baby food jars are ideal for this. You could leave one at work and one in the car, so you're never without your emollient.

Choosing an emollient

The more oil an emollient contains, the better it protects the skin against moisture loss. Ointments typically contain 80 per cent oil and 20 per cent water, whilst creams contain 50 per cent oil and 50 per cent water. Ointments are particularly beneficial in dry, low humidity conditions – for example, in central-heated buildings, or during a spell of cold weather – because the skin loses more moisture in this type of environment. Look for products with petroleum, mineral oil, linoleic acid, or glycerin in the list of ingredients. However, because of their high oil content, ointments can trap sweat next to the skin, causing itchiness, so avoid using them on areas of skin that tend to get hot and sweaty, i.e. the palms of the hands, the soles of the feet and the groin and underarm areas. The effects of oilier products also tend to be more long lasting. They include proprietary emollients such as the Eucerin, Balneum, Oilatum and E45 ranges, all of which are listed in the Useful Products section.

In more humid conditions, the skin can absorb moisture from the air, so a lighter cream or lotion may suffice.

Other moisturising products are mentioned further on in this chapter and in the Useful Products section. The National Eczema Society (details are in the Directory section) provides a more comprehensive Emollient Product List. You could also ask your pharmacist or GP what is available. You may need to try one or two different products until you find one you like that works for you.

Aqueous cream BP
Aqueous cream BP, available on prescription and over-the-counter, is a light emollient, making it useful during the day when a heavier preparation might leave greasy marks. It's quite versatile as it can also be used to wash your hands or body – it cleanses the skin without damaging the delicate skin barrier. However, some people can become sensitised (allergic) to the ingredients, so it tends to be used less often than in the past. A survey carried out by Dr Michael Cork, a skin specialist at Sheffield Children's Hospital, revealed that 56 per cent of children reacted quite badly to aqueous cream (see below).

Emulsifying ointment BP
This heavy emollient, also available on prescription and over the counter, is a mixture of emulsifying wax, white soft paraffin and liquid paraffin. It's particularly good for extremely dry skin that is prone to cracking. However, because of it's heaviness it can cause itchiness in hot conditions, and it is very greasy, which can be a problem when carrying out daytime tasks. As a result of this, it's prescribed less often than in the past.

Skin sensitisers

Many emollients contain ingredients which can cause an allergic skin reaction in some people – these include chemicals which help to extend their shelf life and are often termed 'skin sensitisers'.

Common skin sensitisers include:

- Beeswax, benzyl alcohol and butylated hydroxyanisole

- Butylated hydroxytoluene and cetostearyl alcohol (including cetyl and stearyl alcohol)

- Chlorocresol, edetic acid (EDTA) and ethylenediamine

- Fragrances, hydroxybenzoates (parabens) and imidurea

- Isopropyl palmitate and N-(3-Chloroallyl) hexaminium chloride (quaternium 15)

- Polysorbates and propylene glycol

- Sodium laureth sulphate and sodium metabisulphite

- Sorbic acid and wool fat and associated substances – such as lanolin*

*Some products now contain purified versions of wool fat, which has lessened the problem. However, vegetarians and vegans may prefer to avoid products containing animal derivatives.

Sensitiser-free products

Dr Chris Steele, the resident GP on ITV's *This Morning* programme, claimed recently that many of his patients with eczema have suffered from adverse reactions to emollients – not always immediately, but sometimes over a period of weeks, months or even years. He now tries to prescribe creams that are free of sensitisers. Skincare products for eczema sufferers that are free from sensitisers include the Allergenics, Dermasalve and Salcura ranges, as well as Epaderm. For further information about these products and details of where you can buy them, see the Useful Products section.

> ### Useful tip:
>
> Dr Steele suggests applying emollient, or mild steroid cream, to bad eczema on a limb and then covering it with cling film. This will ensure that all the ointment is absorbed and will speed up healing.

Test it

Because of the risk of an adverse reaction, when trying a new emollient it is advisable to test it out on an eczema-free patch of skin first – for example, on your inner arm. This should be done twice a day for a week, as allergic reactions can sometimes take a while to develop. Only if you are sure your skin has not reacted after this period should you then apply the emollient to the area of your skin affected by eczema.

Sometimes creams or ointments can make your skin itchy and red and even sting a little initially – this is often because of the effect of rubbing the skin during application, or sometimes because the cream prevents sweat escaping from the skin, causing irritation. If these effects settle down within an hour, they are unlikely to be an indicator of an allergic reaction.

Go soap free

Soap can remove the skin's oils and damage the skin barrier, making eczema attacks more likely. Research suggests that the best way to avoid developing eczema is to promote a healthy skin barrier by avoiding the use of harsh soaps and perfumed toiletries during childhood. Instead, try using a water dispersible emollient cream, such as aqueous cream or emulsifying ointment, to wash your hands. For the best results, wash with lukewarm water, rubbing the cream into your hands for a couple of minutes before rinsing away. Use the emollient from a pump dispenser if possible as this reduces the risk of the cream becoming contaminated by bacteria. Remove your rings before washing if you find that trapped moisture triggers your eczema.

3. Try other medications

Tar preparations

Tar is the sticky substance derived from materials like coal and wood and was traditionally used to soothe itchy, inflamed skin. However, it's less popular nowadays because there are less smelly and messy alternatives. It can also be irritating to sore skin. There are also prescription only preparations, such as coal tar solution in one quarter strength Betnovate, where the tar has been mixed with steroid ointments.

Steroid creams

Mild steroid creams help to calm eczema flare-ups by suppressing the body's inflammatory response. The most commonly used steroid cream is hydrocortisone, which is quite mild – 0.1 to 1 per cent – and can be bought over the counter in pharmacies. Creams of this potency are relatively safe when used as directed. Stronger creams have to be prescribed by your GP and should only be used for short periods under supervision. They tend to be prescribed for severe forms of eczema. Generally, the weakest potency that can treat the symptoms effectively should be used. This might involve using a stronger preparation when your symptoms are at their worst and then going on to a milder one as your skin's condition improves. Using excessive amounts for too long can thin the skin, leaving it more fragile.

The British Association of Dermatologists cautions people to use steroid creams sparingly and not to use them as an emollient. Concerns have been raised about using steroid creams on the face because the skin here is thinner and therefore more sensitive. However, Helen Pugsley, dermatology lecturer at Cardiff University, told me, 'one per cent hydrocortisone is safe even for the face and babies and there's no evidence that this strength ever causes any problems'. Stronger versions may lead to cataracts (clouding that develops in the crystalline lens of the eye) or glaucoma (increased pressure in the eye), both of which may affect your vision.

Stopping the use of a steroid cream abruptly may lead to a 'rebound effect', i.e. the eczema flaring up again, so it may be helpful to go on using it for one or two days a week for a week or two after your eczema has settled.

Wet wrapping

Wet wrapping involves the use of an emollient or weak steroid cream together with tubular bandages – it's particularly effective for young eczema sufferers, as it calms inflammation and itching and prevents damage from scratching. First of all an emollient or mild steroid cream is applied to the affected skin. Next, the area is covered with a tubular bandage, which has been soaked in warm water. A dry bandage is then put on, to help keep moisture in and clothing dry. The moisture from the dressing works with the emollient to hydrate the skin and relieve itching. Never cover infected eczema with a wet wrap.

Dry wrapping

This is a similar procedure but a single layer of a dry dressing is used. Its function is mainly to keep the medication in place and prevent scratching and skin damage.

Oral corticosteroids

Strong oral steroids, such as prednisolone, are usually only used for very severe atopic eczema because they have a number of undesirable side effects. They're only available on prescription and work by suppressing the immune system. A course of oral steroids usually lasts between one and four weeks. The dose may be reduced gradually over a few weeks to prevent the risk of a flare-up once the medication is stopped. When oral steroids are taken for a long period of time, the adrenal glands stop producing cortisol, making the body less able to cope with illness, or able to ward off serious illness. The bones also become weakened, leading to an increased risk of osteoporosis in adults and stunted growth among children. Other side effects include mood change, weight gain, thinning of the skin, raised blood pressure and a higher risk of developing diabetes.

Immunomodulatory treatments

These are prescribed as an alternative to steroids – perhaps if they've been ineffective, or if an individual can't tolerate them. Immunomodulators work by changing the body's immune response. The two used for the treatment of eczema are tacrolimus ointment and pimecrolimus cream. In the short term they appear to be safe, but the long-term effects are unknown.

Tacrolimus ointment

Tacrolimus ointment – also known as Protopic – works by dampening down the body's and the skin's immune response, which helps to calm inflammation and reduce itching and redness. It's applied thinly to the skin twice a day and should only be used where there is atopic eczema. It can be used on the skin anywhere on the body except inside the mouth, nose and internal genital area. It can be used alongside an emollient, but it's recommended that these creams are not applied within two hours of each other. Studies suggest that tacrolimus is more effective than weak hydrocortisone creams. The weakest preparation (0.1 per cent) seems to work as well as the stronger hydrocortisone creams. It can offer a solution to severe facial eczema that has not responded to other treatments. Common side effects include a burning sensation, itching and infected hair follicles. However, these effects tend to disappear within a few days. The long-term side effects of using tacrolimus have yet to be established – similar drugs have been linked to an increased risk of skin cancer. With long-term use, excessive sun exposure should be avoided until the effects are known.

Note:

Tacrolimus ointment shouldn't be used where the skin has a viral (e.g. chicken pox, warts or cold sores) or bacterial (e.g. impetigo) infection – it could make them worse, because it reduces the skin's natural resistance. It also shouldn't be used under wet wraps.

Pimecrolimus cream

Pimecrolimus cream works in a similar way to tacrolimus cream, but it's weaker, so it tends to be prescribed for people with mild to moderate eczema. It's also applied twice a day. Pimecrolimus cream can be used alongside emollient, though it can't be mixed and should be applied first. It doesn't cause the skin to thin, so it can be used for the treatment of facial eczema, but it can cause a warm or burning feeling in the areas to which it is applied. This effect tends to be short term. Like tacrolimus, it shouldn't be used under wet wraps and the long-term side effects are as yet unknown.

Note: Both Tacrolimus and Pimecrolimus are unsuitable for use on children under two years.

Antihistamines

Antihistamines are drugs that block the actions of histamines – chemicals produced by the body as part of the allergic response. They can be taken orally in pill, capsule or syrup form, as well as topically in ointments, creams and lotions. Antihistamines have traditionally been prescribed to reduce itching and therefore scratching. There are two types of oral antihistamine – sedating and non-sedating.

Sedating antihistamines cause drowsiness, so they can be useful when itchy skin is preventing sleep. If used over a long period they can become less effective, so they're best used only when acute flare-ups are affecting sleep, in short bursts of no more than two weeks. Helen Pugsley, dermatology lecturer at Cardiff University, explained that non-sedating antihistamines aren't of any benefit unless your eczema is linked to hay fever or urticaria, because the eczema rash itself is not caused by histamine.

Note: Antihistamine creams can sometimes provoke an allergic skin reaction.

Antibiotics
Antibiotics may be prescribed if your eczema becomes infected. But only take them when absolutely necessary, as prolonged use can lead to antibiotic-resistant bacteria.

Note:

For more detailed information and expert advice regarding any of these medications and others that are available for the treatment of eczema, please consult your GP or pharmacist.

4. Try alternative treatments

If you prefer to take a more natural approach, here are some suggestions for alternative skin treatments that could to help soothe your eczema symptoms. Please note, however, that in most cases there is only anecdotal evidence regarding their effectiveness.

Phytosterols

Phytosterols are plant extracts that have similar effects to cortisone. There is limited research regarding their effectiveness, but some sufferers claim they're helpful and view them as a gentler and more natural alternative. Skincare ranges containing phytosterols include Allergenics. For further details see the Useful Products section.

Oat soak

Add oatmeal to your bath to calm inflammation and ease itching. Oats contain avenanthramides, which are both anti-inflammatory and anti-pruritic (anti-itch), as well as moisturising fatty acids and vitamin E. Place a couple of handfuls of oats in a white cotton handkerchief, or a pair of tights, and tie tightly. Either attach the bundle to the bath tap so the water can run through it, or throw it in the bath as it fills. You can even use the bundle as a gentle body puff whilst you're in the bath!

Aloe Aloe!

Aloe vera is a perennial succulent plant that has long been used for its skin moisturising and healing properties. Research suggests that the gel from the plant's leaves has antibacterial and anti-inflammatory effects.

Anecdotally, there's evidence it can relieve the itching and dryness associated with eczema. Some people grow their own aloe vera plants so that they can use the gel directly from the leaf, others prefer to use creams, lotions or gels containing it. Details of aloe vera products, such as Aloe Vera Gelly and Aloe Propolis Creme can be found in the Useful Products section.

Baking soda soother

Some sufferers find relief from itching by adding baking soda to the bath. Use one to two cups in warm, not hot, water. Some people find that applying a paste made from mixing baking powder with a little water can also help.

Calamine cooler

Calamine lotion has been traditionally used to relieve itchy skin. It's especially helpful for rashes that ooze and need to be dried out. Whilst it has a cooling and soothing effect on the skin, it can be too drying, so use it in the short term or mixed with an emollient. Alternatively, buy calamine in a water-based cream or oil-based lotion.

Pansy power

German health authorities recommend an infusion of pansy flowers for the treatment of seborrhoeic eczema, especially in babies. To make an infusion, add one to two teaspoons of fresh flower petals to a cup of boiling water. Allow it to cool and use it as a wet dressing. Pansy flowers contain salicylic acid, which is anti-inflammatory, and saponins and mucilage, which have a softening and soothing action. No adverse effects have been reported when the infusion is applied externally.

Redbush tea

In South Africa, rooibos tea has traditionally been used for its skin-healing properties. It's said to help ease eczema when drunk and also soothe the skin when added to baths. Whilst this may be due to its quercetin content, there is no clinical evidence to back these claims.

Kitchen-cupboard emollient

If you run out of emollient, almost any vegetable oil will do the same job – for example, sunflower or olive oils and even hydrogenated (solid) vegetable oil. Bear in mind, though, that these oils are greasy and have a fairly strong smell – so use them as a last resort.

Witch hazel

One study suggested witch hazel was helpful in reducing inflammation and itching. There's also anecdotal evidence that it helps soothe atopic eczema. It's an astringent and has anti-inflammatory and antibacterial properties, so it can be applied to weeping eczema to promote healing and protect against bacterial infection.

Burdock

Burdock is a traditional herbal medicine that's claimed to have cleansing and purifying properties that can help relieve skin eruptions and soothe inflammation. It's also thought to contain inulin, a prebiotic which helps to normalise the immune system by stimulating the growth of good bacteria in the gut. There's no clinical evidence to back up these claims.

Calendula and chamomile

The integrated health expert Dr Andrew Weil, like many alternative health practitioners, recommends the use of creams containing chamomile or calendula. They're thought to have anti-inflammatory properties that soothe the skin and promote healing.

St John's Wort

This herb is most often used for the treatment of depression, but it's also been traditionally used topically (i.e. directly onto the skin) for skin complaints, including eczema. It contains a substance called hypericin that's believed to have anti-inflammatory properties. In a double-blind study, a cream containing St John's Wort extract was compared against a placebo cream among 21 people with mild to moderate eczema. In the study, participants used the St John's Wort cream on one arm and the placebo cream on the other. The results suggested that the use of St John's Wort cream significantly reduced eczema symptoms.

5. Prepare for the sun

Some people find their eczema improves when they're on holiday – especially those with allergic contact dermatitis or discoid eczema. Apart from the fact that people tend to be more relaxed, it's thought that the sun's rays can be beneficial – ultraviolet light is sometimes used in the treatment of eczema. It's believed to work by suppressing the immune response.

However, it's still important to use sunblock to protect the skin from the harmful effects of UVA (long wave solar radiation) and UVB (medium wave solar radiation) rays.

Other people might find that the sun causes, or exacerbates, their eczema. This is known as photosensitive (or light sensitive) eczema. Some drugs, chemicals and herbs can increase the skin's sensitivity to sunlight, e.g. antihistamines, antibiotics and St John's Wort. See your GP if you're affected.

Selecting a suncream

Not all sunscreens protect against UVA, so read the label before buying. Choose one that states it protects against both UVA and UVB rays. These are sometimes labelled 'broad spectrum'. The sun protection factor (SPF) shows how much protection the suncream gives against UVB radiation. The British Association of Dermatology recommends a factor 30 plus to allow for the fact that most of us don't apply enough sunscreen. This level of protection allows only 4 per cent of UVB rays to get through. Higher factors offer more protection – e.g. factor 60 allows only 2 per cent of UVB rays to get through.

UVA protection is indicated by nought to five stars – though this is just a rough guide because it is also affected by the SPF. For example, a cream with SPF 25 and three stars might give more UVA protection overall than a cream with SPF 10 and four stars. Waterproof cream is less likely to be washed or sweated off. Also, some of the greasier suncreams may trap perspiration on the skin and cause irritation.

As is the case when choosing emollients, checking the labels can help you to avoid substances you have a known sensitivity to. Sunscreens are chemical, or mineral based, or a combination of the two. Chemical creams are absorbed into the skin, whilst mineral-based creams stay on the skin's surface, forming a reflective barrier. The chemicals can irritate the skin and cause sensitivity, so eczema sufferers may find mineral based creams more suitable. The mineral used is usually titanium dioxide. Suitable suncream ranges for eczema sufferers include Uvistat Suncare and E45 Suncare. For further details, including stockists, see the Useful Products section.

Slap it on!

It is advisable to test a cream for adverse reactions by applying it to a small area of skin first, before using it on your whole body.

Cancer Research UK advises people to put suncream on before going out in the sun and before applying emollient or moisturiser, so it's next to the skin. Apply it thickly, or as the Australians say, 'Slap it on' for maximum benefit and then repeat to ensure you haven't missed anywhere. Reapply your suncream at least every two hours and immediately after swimming or heavy perspiration. Don't rub it in too well, or you'll lose some protection. Exposure to the sun is drying for your skin, so it's a good idea to use more emollient than usual and perhaps a richer one at night.

Stay safe

You can still burn whilst wearing suncream, so keep an eye on your skin all the time – especially children's skin, which is more delicate. Avoid the sun's rays between 11 a.m. and 3 p.m., as this is when they are at their strongest. Cover up – wear a hat and sunglasses or stay in the shade – but remember the sun's rays reflect off water, sand and snow, so continue to wear suncream. Wearing cotton or linen clothing will not only protect your skin against the sun, it will also help you to stay cool. Some people find that overheating can trigger their eczema, or the sweating it causes can exacerbate itching.

6. Take care of your skin in the water

In the swim

Swimming is relaxing and good for increasing fitness. However, whether you swim in the sea or a pool you may find it worsens your eczema symptoms. Like seawater, the water in swimming pools can aggravate eczema. This is because it contains chlorine, which is an irritant. If you're affected, try using a light emollient such as aqueous cream on your skin before you enter the pool. Shower yourself thoroughly when you get out and reapply the emollient. Jacuzzis tend to contain a much higher concentration of chemicals.

Some people notice an improvement in their eczema after swimming. Helen Pugsley, dermatology lecturer at Cardiff University, told me that this may be because chlorine has an antibacterial effect on the skin.

On the beach

Seawater and sand can be irritating to some eczema sufferers, especially if the skin is cracked or broken and particles get trapped, causing stinging. Applying a light emollient can help to protect against these effects. A heavy emollient might make the skin overheat and itch.

After a trip to the beach, a lukewarm bath or shower will remove salt and sand. Apply an emollient afterwards to soothe the skin. On the other hand, some people find seawater improves their eczema. This may be due to the salt in the water having an antiseptic effect.

Take to the tub

Soaking in the bath can be beneficial because the water moisturises the skin's outer layer as well as removing dirt and bacteria. It can also help to remove crusts from the skin during a flare-up. Lukewarm water is best, as hot water may dry out or irritate the skin. Use emollient in the bath instead of foam bath, which contains detergent that can damage your skin's protective barrier. Many of the proprietary ranges for dry skin include special shower and bath emollients – see Useful Products.

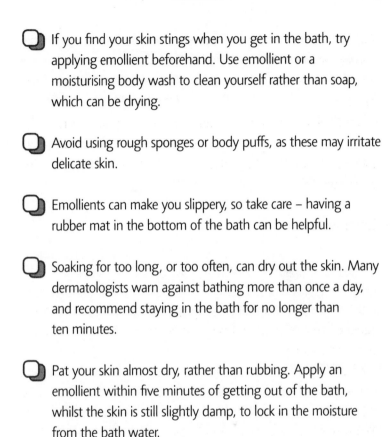

If you find your skin stings when you get in the bath, try applying emollient beforehand. Use emollient or a moisturising body wash to clean yourself rather than soap, which can be drying.

Avoid using rough sponges or body puffs, as these may irritate delicate skin.

Emollients can make you slippery, so take care – having a rubber mat in the bottom of the bath can be helpful.

Soaking for too long, or too often, can dry out the skin. Many dermatologists warn against bathing more than once a day, and recommend staying in the bath for no longer than ten minutes.

Pat your skin almost dry, rather than rubbing. Apply an emollient within five minutes of getting out of the bath, whilst the skin is still slightly damp, to lock in the moisture from the bath water.

7. Dress sensibly

What you wear can have an effect on your eczema. Wool and synthetic fibres can cause irritation. Cotton or cotton mixes seem to work best because they keep the skin cool and allow it to breathe. Avoid wearing tight, constrictive clothes as they can rub the skin or cause sweating, which can exacerbate both atopic and dyshydrotic eczema. There are details of cotton clothing stockists in the Useful Products section. Some people find that the detergent they use to wash their clothes with can irritate their skin – see 40. 'Use non-biological washing powders' in Chapter 5 for details.

8. Identify when you scratch

A survey of 440 eczema sufferers by the National Eczema Society revealed that they viewed itching as the worst aspect of their condition. Eighty-five per cent of respondents said it affected their sleep, 62 per cent said it affected their work and 58 per cent said it interfered with their social life.

Ditch that itch

The skincare tips mentioned so far should help to relieve the itch of eczema; however, other factors may be involved. An important step in reducing itching is to identify when and why you itch. So if you're using emollients regularly but still find your skin is itchy you need to pinpoint what makes the itch worse. Are you using the wrong type of emollient? Remember, you need different types for different environments. For a week, make a note of when your skin itches the most. Is the itching more troublesome during the day? Perhaps your clothing is scratching your skin? Does it tend to be worse at night? Could your bedding be irritating your skin, or is the atmosphere in your bedroom too hot, or too dry? For more ideas on what could be exacerbating your itching, e.g. the chemicals in household cleaners, see Chapter 4 – Home Front. Once you've taken steps to reduce the itch, you can focus your attention on resisting the urge to scratch.

The scratching habit

The natural response to an itch is to scratch it – unfortunately, scratching makes eczema worse by causing the release of histamine, a chemical implicated in allergic reactions. This in turn increases the itching, leading to further scratching and damage to the epidermis, including possibly breaking the skin, which leaves the skin open to infection and increased inflammation. This leads to more itching and scratching – a vicious circle. In cases of chronic eczema the scratching has often become a habit. Dermatologists and psychiatrists at the Chelsea and Westminster Hospital conducted research which suggested that emollients and steroids were of little use if patients continued to scratch. They developed a programme to help their patients with eczema break their scratching habit. The programme helps eczema sufferers become aware of when and how they scratch and then suggests techniques to help them break and replace their scratching habit. Some people find it can help them control their eczema symptoms when used in conjunction with emollients and steroid creams.

The first step to breaking your scratching habit is to become aware of when, where, why and how you scratch. Carry a notepad and pen around with you and record: the time of day; where you are; how you scratch and why. For example, one study claims that many sufferers scratch whilst watching television. You may notice you scratch first thing in the morning, when you arrive home after work or at bedtime when you're feeling tired. Do you tend to scratch in response to an itch, or is it just out of habit a lot of the time? Scratching includes rubbing, scraping with, or against, something and picking. By noting down these details you should be able to pinpoint your 'danger times' when you're more likely to scratch. You can then plan activities to help you deal with these periods. For example, if you tend to scratch when you arrive home after a stressful day at work, aim at doing something relaxing when you first get home – like listening to music or having a relaxing soak in the bath.

Sample scratch record

When did you scratch?				
Where were you?				
Why did you scratch?				
How did you scratch?				

9. Stop scratching

The Chelsea and Westminster Programme suggests that every time you get the urge to scratch you should clench your fists gently for around 30 seconds, whilst thinking about something pleasant and calming. I find imagining myself lying on a golden beach with glorious blue skies and the sound of waves lapping takes my mind off the itch totally! If the area is still itching when you reach 30 seconds, press a fingernail – preferably a short one – into the area, or gently pinch the skin. This helps to relieve the itch and is less damaging than scratching. If the fist clenching and visualisation is enough to stop the scratching urge, you don't need to go on to the pressing or pinching stage.

The idea is that clenching your fists and thinking pleasant thoughts helps you to stop scratching out of habit, whilst pressing or pinching helps you to control scratching in response to itching.

A review of interventions for atopic eczema in 2000 concluded that habit-reversal techniques like this are useful when combined with other treatments e.g. emollients and/or steroids. The Chelsea and Westminster six-week programme is outlined in a book called *The Eczema Solution*. For further details see the Helpful Books section.

Damage limitation

Whilst you're trying to reduce the itch and the urge to scratch you can also take practical steps to reduce the damage to your skin that your scratching causes. Keeping nails as short as possible is a simple way to limit harm from scratching. For children, putting on cotton mittens at bedtime can help lessen the effects of scratching during the night.

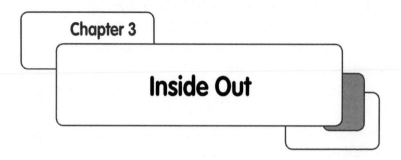

Chapter 3

Inside Out

This chapter looks at how the food you eat may be implicated in your eczema symptoms. A balanced diet is important for general health and could improve your eczema – particularly if it's linked to deficiencies of particular nutrients such as vitamins A, B complex, C and E, zinc and essential fatty acids. It will also cover supplements commonly suggested for the treatment of eczema and whether their use is supported by scientific research or anecdotal evidence.

Some people believe that food allergies and intolerances and even yeast infections such as candida, caused by eating particular foods, are linked to eczema. The foods most commonly implicated – e.g. wheat, dairy, peanuts and sugar – will be explained in this chapter. However, the idea that excluding particular foods from the diet can improve eczema symptoms is controversial, so I have also included expert opinions and the important points to bear in mind should you decide to make dietary changes.

10. Keep your skin well hydrated

Drinking plenty of water is vital for well-being and healthy skin. Keep your skin well hydrated by drinking plenty of fluids – ideally around 2 litres of water a day.

Some waters from particular areas are believed to offer specific health benefits. Lakeland Willow Spring water is high in salicin, an anti-inflammatory, and is claimed to help clear up eczema. Kate Murray, an eczema sufferer from Hampshire, claims she found relief from her eczema for the first time in ten years when she started drinking Lakeland Willow Water. A local vet had recommended it for her puppy's skin problems! However, the evidence is strictly anecdotal – as yet there is no clinical evidence to back up these claims.

11. Nourish your skin with a balanced diet

If you suffer from eczema it's especially important to eat well to keep yourself healthy and help prevent flare-ups. A balanced diet is one that consists of around one-third fruit and vegetables and one-third unrefined carbohydrates, like wholemeal bread, brown pasta and rice, and potatoes cooked in their skins. The remaining third should comprise roughly equal amounts of protein foods like fish, poultry and lean meat and low-fat dairy foods like yogurt and cheese, with a small amount of sugar and fatty foods.

Fruit and vegetables supply vitamins, minerals and fibre, as well as plant nutrients, which appear to actively ward off disease. They also contain the antioxidants vitamins A, C and E, which are believed to protect the skin from damage from the sun and pollutants. Quercetin – a plant nutrient found in fruit and vegetables such as apples and onions – is thought to reduce the allergic response.

Healthy eating is about getting the balance right. You can still eat fatty and sugary foods – so long as you view them as a treat and eat them sparingly.

A balanced diet will help to ensure you obtain the nutrients you need for healthy skin. These include vitamins A, B complex, C and E and the mineral zinc. Research suggests it's best to obtain these from your diet as much as possible.

Vitamin A

Vitamin A is an antioxidant. Antioxidants neutralise the skin-ageing free radicals the body produces when we are stressed or exposed to sunlight and pollutants such as cigarette smoke, chemicals and food additives. Vitamin A is also essential for your skin's growth and repair, as well as helping to counter infections, ease allergy symptoms and boost moisture retention.

This vitamin comes in two forms – retinol and beta-carotene. Retinol is found in animal products such as liver, fish-liver oils, egg yolks, whole milk, cheese and butter. Beta-carotene is found in plants – especially in yellow and orange fruits and vegetables such as carrots, sweet potatoes, butternut squash, cantaloupe melons, orange and yellow peppers and apricots.

Vitamin B complex

Adequate amounts of vitamin B complex are essential for healthy skin. A lack of some B vitamins – especially biotin and vitamin B6 – is thought to contribute to eczema, including seborrhoeic eczema.

Good sources of vitamin B complex include wholegrains, nuts, seeds, wheatgerm, meat (especially liver), fish and eggs.

Vitamin C

Vitamin C also has an antioxidant effect and is essential for the production of collagen, the main protein in your skin that gives it strength, elasticity and moisture. It also has antihistamine properties and helps to combat skin infections.

Vitamin C is found in fruit and vegetables – especially citrus fruits, blackcurrants, berries, peppers, broccoli and cabbage.

Vitamin E

Vitamin E is also an antioxidant and helps to keep your skin soft and smooth. In one study, 50 per cent of the participants taking vitamin E supplements had far less eczema after eight months, whilst only 2 per cent who took a placebo reported that their eczema had improved. Fifteen per cent of those who took the supplements claimed their eczema cleared up completely. A short Japanese study showed that vitamin E combined with vitamin B2 was more effective in reducing eczema than when either were taken alone. However, the results were deemed inconclusive, because there wasn't a control group taking a placebo to compare the outcomes with. Other studies have found that vitamin E doesn't help people with eczema, but it may still be worth trying as part of your eczema prevention programme.

Vitamin E is found in nuts and seeds, avocados, sweet potatoes, olive oil and wheatgerm.

Zinc

Zinc is an important mineral for the protection, maintenance, defence and healing of the skin. It's thought that a shortage may affect the metabolism of fatty acids and therefore contribute to eczema symptoms. One clinical trial failed to show that zinc supplementation benefits atopic eczema, though.

Zinc is found in meat, shellfish, bread, wholegrain cereals, beans, lentils, nuts, seeds and dairy products such as cheese and milk.

Essential fatty acids

Essential fatty acids (EFAs) are fats that can't be produced by the body and are needed for various functions, including healthy skin.

Research suggests that some eczema sufferers may have a deficiency in essential fatty acids, or have problems metabolising them. Ensuring you eat foods or take supplements which supply them, may help to reduce your symptoms.

Omega-3s are anti-inflammatory and are believed to help protect against skin complaints, as well as many common diseases, including cardiovascular disease and arthritis. Good sources of omega-3s include oily fish – pilchards, sardines, salmon and mackerel; nuts – especially walnuts, Brazil nuts and almonds; seeds – especially sesame; oils, including hemp seed, soya bean, sunflower, canola and rapeseed; and egg yolks.

Omega-6s are also anti-inflammatory and may help prevent and treat a range of conditions as well as promote healthy skin. Gamma linoleic acid is a type of omega-6 fatty acid. One of the best-known sources is evening primrose oil. Omega-6 fatty acids are also found in sunflower, olive and corn oils, olives, nuts, seeds and some vegetables and grains.

Ex-seedingly good snacks

Instead of snacking on crisps or biscuits, try a handful of seeds such as sunflower, sesame or pumpkin. As well as EFAs they contain iron, zinc, calcium and magnesium.

12. Supplement your diet

If you find it difficult to eat a balanced diet, for whatever reason, supplements can help to safeguard against nutritional deficiencies. Supplements are controversial, with some recent reports claiming that isolated substances don't provide the same benefits that nutrients found in foods do. However, for many of us, supplements represent a convenient means of improving our diets. Some over-the-counter products are unregistered. This means there's no guarantee of their content and quality. Once EU legislation has come into force in April 2011, safety levels will be higher. In the meantime, always buy products from a reputable company – if in doubt, ask your GP or pharmacist.

Sometimes there's no scientific evidence to back up these claims. This doesn't necessarily mean a substance is ineffective or unsafe – it's often simply because the research hasn't been done.

Evening primrose oil

Rich in gamma linoleic acid, an omega-6 fatty acid, evening primrose oil, derived from a flowering plant found in North and South America, has been recommended for the treatment and prevention of eczema since the 1930s. The gamma linoleic acid is thought to block the pathway of chemical messengers known as prostaglandins, which are linked to inflammation and itching. The evidence is conflicting, with some studies reporting no benefits and others suggesting a small improvement – especially in terms of reducing itching. However, this supplement may be worth taking for three months, to see whether you are one of those people who can benefit from it. It appears to be safe when taken as recommended by the manufacturer, but people with epilepsy shouldn't take it, as it may increase the risk of fits. High doses of 6 to 8 g daily are needed, but Helen Pugsley, dermatology lecturer at Cardiff University, cautioned that this 'is a problem for small children'. The recommended dose for children is 2 to 4 g.

Fish oils
Fish oils contain omega-3 fatty acids, and supplements are often recommended as beneficial for eczema sufferers; however, there's little evidence that they work. One study in 1989 suggested that taking 10 g of fish oil daily reduces eczema symptoms, including itching and scales. The researchers claimed that the fish oils worked by reducing levels of an inflammatory substance called leukotriene B4, which is linked to eczema.

Subsequent reviews have concluded that there's insufficient good evidence that it benefits the condition. However, this supplement may still be worth trying – it's believed to benefit physical and mental health as well.

Liquorice
Liquorice is used by many herbalists for the treatment of eczema. It contains glycyrrhetinic acid, which is thought to relieve itching and inflammation. It's often included in Chinese herbal preparations, which are becoming more popular in the treatment of eczema. As well as taking liquorice internally, creams containing glycyrrhetinic acid from liquorice may be helpful in relieving itching. There's anecdotal, but no scientific, evidence to back up these claims.

Chamomile tea
Chamomile tea has traditionally been drunk to ease various health problems, including dermatitis. It's also thought to have anti-inflammatory properties. There's only anecdotal evidence that it works.

Chinese cure?

Recent research from Hong Kong, published in the British Journal of Dermatology', concluded that a concoction of herbs used by the Chinese for thousands of years could ease eczema. The mixture included Japanese honeysuckle, peppermint, root bark of tree peony, underground stem of the atractylodes herb and bark from an Amur cork tree. Eczema sufferers aged from five to 21 reported dramatic improvement in their symptoms and a reduction in their need for conventional treatments, such as steroids.

Nina Goad of the British Association of Dermatologists commented: 'These early studies show that children with atopic eczema may benefit from a specific concoction of traditional Chinese herbs, which could eventually pave the way for this remedy to find its way into mainstream medicine. However, we would warn against using Chinese herbal medications without first speaking to your doctor. Some retailers may not be reputable and the product they sell you may be of a low standard or could contain harmful ingredients.'

13. Identify your food allergies

Some people claim that their eczema is due to a food sensitivity and find relief when they avoid what they believe are the offending items. Food sensitivity is complex, but in simple terms there are two main forms: immediate and delayed.

Immediate sensitivity

In immediate food sensitivity, symptoms such as itching develop within an hour or two of eating the food. Other common signs are redness, irritation and swelling around the mouth, eczema, urticaria, itchy eyes, stomach pain, muscle weakness, vomiting, wheezing and sneezing. This is a true allergy, as it involves the immune system. Where the reaction is severe, it's known as anaphylaxis. Here symptoms are more pronounced and there may be swelling of the lips, mouth and tongue. In extreme cases, there can be a sudden drop in blood pressure and loss of consciousness – anaphylactic shock – which can lead to death.

Some researchers believe that people who react in this way to certain foods may have a leaky gut wall. This is where it becomes over-permeable, possibly due to stress or irritants such as coffee, alcohol or some medications. In this state it allows molecules of food to enter the bloodstream, where they trigger the immune response.

Always call an ambulance immediately if you suspect an anaphylactic reaction. If you experience the milder symptoms of food sensitivity, consult your GP as soon as possible.

Delayed sensitivity

In delayed sensitivity, symptoms such as increased itching and eczema appear within six to 24 hours of eating the trigger food. There may also be stomach pain and diarrhoea. This isn't a true allergy, as it doesn't involve the immune response and is more likely to be due to an intolerance, otherwise known as non-allergic hypersensitivity.

If you're atopic, you're at risk of suffering from both immediate and delayed food sensitivity.

Common culprits

The foods most commonly implicated in immediate food sensitivity are usually proteins, found in foods such as wheat, milk and peanuts. Even tiny amounts can set off an allergic reaction. This type of food sensitivity appears to be most common in babies and young children and generally disappears by the age of five.

The foods often linked to delayed food sensitivity are likely to be food staples, so wheat and milk are the common causes in the western world. In Asia, people are more likely to be sensitive to rice.

Common culprits include grains (wheat, rye, oats and corn), dairy products (milk, cheese and hens' eggs). Peanuts, tree nuts (almonds, hazelnuts, pecans and walnuts), beef, poultry, pork, white fish, shellfish (e.g. prawns), citrus fruits, bananas, chocolate and soya can also be responsible for food sensitive reactions. Other items that have been known to trigger a reaction include tea, coffee, alcohol, yeast and food additives.

Wheat sensitivity

Wheat allergy is thought to be relatively uncommon. One of the prime allergens in wheat is a protein called gliadin, which is found in gluten. This is why people with a wheat allergy are sometimes advised to eat a gluten-free diet.

That said, wheat allergy and coeliac disease are different conditions, and foods that are labelled as being 'gluten free' may not be suitable for people with a wheat allergy.

Since November 2005, food-labelling legislation requires pre-packed foods sold in the UK, and the rest of the EU, to indicate on the label if they include cereals containing gluten, such as wheat, rye, barley and oats.

If you believe that you have a wheat allergy or intolerance that is causing, or exacerbating, your eczema, you should see your GP or other health professional before changing your diet.

Dairy food sensitivity

Dairy foods are believed to be one of the most common causes of food intolerances among eczema sufferers. Dairy intolerance can be due to an inability to break down lactose – milk sugar – hence the phrase 'lactose intolerance', or an allergic response to milk proteins.

Experts are divided over whether eliminating dairy from the diet is beneficial or not. Some eczema sufferers or parents of children with eczema have claimed that doing so has reduced symptoms.

Only follow a diet free of dairy products if a reliable test has shown that you or your child have an allergy or intolerance. Dairy foods supply essential nutrients such as calcium – eliminating them from your diet could cause other health problems, including insomnia and osteoporosis and growth problems in children, unless alternative sources are eaten. These include dark green leafy vegetables, sardines – including the bones – almonds, Brazil nuts, seeds, dried apricots, figs, dates, lentils and beans. Make sure you follow the advice of your GP or dietician. Following a dairy free diet requires discipline and determination. You will need to read food labels because milk and milk products are used in many processed foods. The word 'milk' comes in many guises – whey, casein, caseinates, lactalbumin and lactose are all derived from milk. Cooking your own meals from scratch may help. Most supermarkets now stock dairy-free products, for example those containing soya and goat's milk and cheese, which appear to cause fewer adverse reactions. Some people who can't tolerate milk find they can eat natural yogurt without any problems. It's thought that the bacteria they contain breaks down the milk proteins, making them easier to digest.

Peanut sensitivity

Peanuts are sometimes known as groundnuts or monkey nuts. If someone is allergic to peanuts they usually are for life. However, research indicates that, in a very few cases, children diagnosed with peanut allergy can sometimes grow out of it.

Peanuts are one of the commonest causes of food allergy and can cause reactions ranging from atopic eczema to anaphylaxis. They contain various allergens that aren't destroyed by cooking. Roasting peanuts actually makes them more likely to cause an allergic reaction. Even tiny amounts of peanut can cause a reaction in individuals who are sensitive. For example, eating food containing minute traces of peanuts or even just being near someone eating peanuts can be enough to cause a reaction in some individuals. Peanuts are sometimes used instead of pine nuts in food products like pesto, so those who are allergic to peanuts should be careful when eating foods usually made with pine nuts. Since November 2005, food labelling legislation has required manufacturers of pre-packed food sold in the UK, and the rest of the EU, to indicate clearly on the label if the product contains peanuts – or if one of its ingredients contains them.

Health professionals generally agree that refined peanut oil is unlikely to cause problems for people with peanut allergy, because almost all the proteins that cause allergic reactions tend to be removed during manufacturing. But refined peanut oil is still included in the revised food-labelling rules, so it's listed as 'peanut oil' when used in pre-packaged foods.

Cold-pressed, or unrefined, peanut oil may contain peanut proteins, which can provoke a reaction in peanut-sensitive individuals. Peanut oil is sometimes known as 'groundnut oil'.

Some individuals with a peanut allergy may also react to legumes like soya, green beans, kidney beans, green peas and the lupin plant, because these foods contain allergens similar to those found in peanuts. People with a peanut allergy can sometimes also be allergic to nuts such as almonds, Brazil nuts, cashew nuts, pecans, hazelnuts and walnuts.

14. Be aware of food additives

Some experts think that the greater incidence of eczema is down to the increased use of food additives. According to the Food Standards Agency, studies have shown that foods containing E102 Tartrazine may trigger eczema in some people. Anecdotal evidence links some other food dyes to skin rashes, despite them being deemed safe by the EU (hence the E number). These include:

E104 Quinoline yellow
E110 Sunset yellow
E122 Carmoisine
E123 Amaranth
E124 Ponceau
E128 Red 2G
E155 Brown HT

Certain preservatives are thought to irritate the skin and thus could make eczema symptoms worse. These include:

E200 Sorbic acid
E216 Propyl p-hydroxybenzoate

E217 Sodium propyl p-hydroxybenzoate

E218 Methyl p-hydroxybenzoate

E219 Sodium methyl p-hydroxybenzoate

15. Eat the right foods during pregnancy and childhood

Beneficial bugs

A small study in 2001 found that children who took probiotics twice a day were more likely to report their eczema symptoms were improving than those who took a placebo treatment. The supplements used in this study contained the bacteria called *Lactobacillus rhamnosus* and *Lactobacillus reuteri*.

In another much larger study in 2006 involving 1,223 women in their last month of pregnancy, half were given a probiotic mixture containing *Lactobacilli* and *Bifidobacteria*, and the other half were given a placebo. The children were then given either the mixture or the placebo for six months. The results showed that the probiotic mixture reduced the incidence of eczema.

A study in 2008 had similar results. Some experts believe that the increase in allergies is due to people not being exposed to bacteria during childhood. This is thought to be partly due to the fact we no longer eat unpasteurised foods, which stimulated the immune system. It's thought that probiotics have a similar effect. More research is needed, but in the meantime it may be worth including probiotics such as natural yogurt in your diet, especially when pregnant. Encourage your children to eat it too. There are several types available – I find natural set bio-yogurt delicious on its own or with fresh fruit, or as a replacement for sour cream in Mexican dishes like chilli con carne. Some children may find the flavour too acidic – try adding honey to sweeten it. If you prefer to take a supplement try ProbioStart or Vinalac Probiotic Formula, both of which are specifically formulated for pregnant and breastfeeding women. Further details are in the Useful Products section.

Breast is best!

If allergies run in your family and you're concerned your child may be at risk, breastfeeding is recommended for the first four to six months. Breast milk is nutritionally superior to cow's milk – it's designed for babies and contains the correct balance of nutrients, antibodies, hormones and antioxidants babies need to thrive. It's also much easier to digest than cow's milk and allows the infant's digestive system to prepare for the introduction of solid foods, making intolerances and allergies less likely to develop.

If you aren't able to breastfeed, or choose not to, there are hydrolyzed formulas in which the proteins are broken down, so that they are more easily digested than normal preparations and help reduce the risk of allergies and intolerances. Some research suggests that baby milk formulas containing prebiotics may reduce the risk of developing eczema.

Delay solids

Because food allergy is especially linked with atopic eczema in children, experts recommend delaying the introduction of solids until the age of four to six months to lessen the risk. Avoid introducing common food triggers, such as cow's milk, eggs, wheat, peanuts, citrus fruits, fish and chocolate until the age of at least six to nine months or even up to a year. Try not to give your child peanuts until at least the age of four. It's also a good idea to introduce new foods one at a time and to wait for a day or two, in case your baby shows signs of a reaction. All of these points are especially important if there is a family history of allergies.

What the experts say

The idea that some foods can cause eczema is controversial. A recent survey of 100 eczema sufferers at Leicester Royal Infirmary revealed that although almost a third had tried excluding foods such as dairy, wheat, alcohol, eggs and tomatoes, 80 per cent felt there had been no improvement in their skin's condition. As a result, dermatologists at the Royal Infirmary warned eczema sufferers against making dietary changes without first consulting their GP.

According to The British Association of Dermatologists, atopic people are more likely to suffer from food allergy, but it's rare for such allergies to cause eczema. They advise people with eczema to focus on eating a healthy, well-balanced diet.

Helen Pugsley, dermatology lecturer at Cardiff University, told me, 'There are five big food groups known to exacerbate eczema, but there is no clinical evidence that exclusion diets work for eczema.'

Recent research has shown that hydrocortisone creams and emollients can often clear up eczema without the need to resort to exclusion diets. Experts recommend that such diets should only be attempted when other therapies have failed to bring relief.

Nutritional therapists' views

Nutritional consultant Patrick Holford advocates detecting and eliminating allergens. He suggests the most common culprits are milk, eggs and peanuts. He also advises eating wholegrains, fresh fruit and vegetables and oily fish, whilst avoiding processed, refined and sugary foods and limiting red meat, dairy and fried foods. In addition, he recommends taking a good multivitamin and mineral supplement to boost your immune system and provide the nutrients needed to heal your skin and an essential fatty acid supplement. He believes that although such a dietary plan may take a while to work, it will bring longer lasting relief.

Dr Andrew Weil, expert in integrated medicine, and Ian Marber, 'The Food Doctor', offer similar advice. Weil explains that processed foods – especially those containing hydrogenated fats or polyunsaturated vegetable oils – and sugary foods increase inflammation. Marber suggests that refined carbohydrates, including sugary foods, can disrupt the metabolism of essential fatty acids which, as we've already noted, can be a problem for people with atopic eczema.

Holford, Weil and Marber all recommend probiotics daily to encourage healthy bacteria in the gut – this could be as a supplement, or as natural bio-yogurt.

16. Learn from others' experiences with food

Kathleen Waterford's story

Kathleen Waterford is an eczema sufferer who believes that a yeast infection – candida – was responsible for her severe eczema. She claims that following a natural 'caveman' type diet – i.e. one that consists of poultry, fish, a little beef, non legume vegetables, nuts, seeds and olive oil, and avoids sugar, dairy foods and grains – has cured her symptoms. Incidentally, Kathleen does suggest the reintroduction of certain starchy foods, such as brown rice and potatoes, after five weeks of following her initial recommendations, which makes the diet slightly more balanced. Whilst this diet seems extreme and shouldn't be undertaken without consulting your GP first, it may be worth a try if all else has failed. The 'caveman' diet is more balanced than it first appears – although it excludes dairy foods, which are rich in bone-building calcium, it includes other sources, such as leafy green vegetables, nuts and seeds.

Details of Kathleen's book, *The Skin Cure Diet*, in which she outlines her experiences and the diet she follows, can be found in the Helpful Books section at the end of this book.

What is candida?

Candida is a type of yeast that can be found in dark, moist areas of the body including the mouth, the digestive and genito-urinary tracts, as well as on the skin. It's thought that healthy bacteria control the number of yeasts in the gut, but if the immune system is depleted, a sugary diet is eaten, or there are insufficient 'good' bacteria in the gut, candida can grow out of control and have a detrimental effect on an individual's health. Common symptoms include thrush and some people believe eczema may also be caused by candida. However, the medical profession is generally sceptical of these claims. The Henry Spink Foundation offers more detailed information and links. Contact details are in the Directory section.

Jennifer Worth's story

Jennifer Worth, a former nursing sister and best-selling author of *Call the Midwife*, also suffered from debilitating eczema, for which she tried every type of treatment imaginable – including steroid creams, spiritual healing, homeopathy, aromatherapy, hypnotherapy and Chinese herbalism.

After two years of suffering from severe eczema all over her body, she met a doctor who was a member of the British Society for Allergy and Environmental and Nutritional Medicine and an allergy sufferer himself. He was an expert in allergy related conditions and had treated eczema sufferers successfully. After telling him that her skin had once improved when she'd had a stomach bug and not eaten for four days, he told her that once they found the right diet for her, her skin would begin to clear.

Jennifer then followed an elimination diet consisting of fresh meats, root vegetables, green vegetables, rice, olive oil, salt and spring water. After trying various food combinations, it turned out that she was allergic to rice and onions. She gradually re-introduced foods and discovered that several, including apples, pears, bananas and fish, triggered her eczema. Eventually, Jennifer's GP agreed to refer her to have a desensitising treatment, which enabled her to eat more foods without her skin reacting. According to Jennifer, Enzyme Potentiated Desensitisation is available on the NHS, via GP referral, at the Royal London Homeopathic Hospital, Great Ormond Street, London (see Directory). Private referrals can be made by a doctor, or by patients themselves. It seems that Jennifer's case was very unusual and extreme and she isn't sure what caused her body to react so badly to so many everyday foods. However, she believes food intolerance may be the hidden cause of some people's eczema. Details of her book, *Eczema and Food Allergy – The Hidden Cause?* can be found in the Helpful Books Section.

17. Keep a food diary

Whilst I have included information about food intolerances and cases studies where they have been shown to cause eczema, the expert view is that anyone suffering from eczema shouldn't automatically assume that their condition is due to a food intolerance. For many people, eating a balanced diet and following a healthy lifestyle will lead to healthier skin.

However, if your eczema still persists, it may then be worth keeping a food diary to determine whether there is a link between what you eat and your symptoms. An ordinary notebook will do – simply note down every food you eat and any symptoms, such as increased itching, redness or swelling, stomach pain, diarrhoea, nausea, problems sleeping etc., each day for four to six weeks. You may see a pattern emerging. If your findings confirm your suspicions, your next step should be to visit your GP, armed with this information.

18. Take a skin test

There are several allergy tests – the first two can be performed by your GP.

Skin prick test

This test is useful for diagnosing immediate food sensitivity. A few drops of extract of the suspect food/s are applied to the skin – usually the forearm – then a small prick or scratch is made. If the area reacts by becoming red and itchy, it confirms sensitivity. Some experts claim that the test is unreliable because of difficulties in interpreting the results. Also, because the skin of eczema sufferers is so sensitive, the scratching itself may trigger a reaction, rather than the substance. However, a positive result suggests that food sensitivity is a possibility. This test can also be used to identify allergies to other substances such as house dust mites, animal dander, pollens and mould. Where there has been an anaphylactic reaction to a specific allergen, skin testing may not be appropriate or necessary.

RAST test

Another test that is used to detect food sensitivity is RAST (Radio Allergo Sorbent Test) – otherwise known as the IgE antibody test. This measures the level of antibodies in the blood following intake of the suspected food. As this measures IgE levels, it's an indicator of immediate food sensitivity – a true allergic reaction involving the immune system. It doesn't reveal delayed food sensitivity, because this doesn't involve the production of antibodies. If a high level of antibodies is detected, it suggests the ingested food could be causing a reaction. This test can give the wrong results and can only test for the common allergens, such as peanuts and eggs.

Exclusion and challenge test

If the results of either test point to a food sensitivity, your GP may refer you to a dietician who may suggest following an 'exclusion and challenge test' which involves stopping eating the suspect food/foods for two to six weeks to see if your symptoms improve. You'll then be asked to reintroduce the food/foods to see if your eczema worsens again. Finally, you'll be asked to exclude the suspected foods to see if the eczema clears up again. It's best to carry out this process under the supervision of your GP and a dietician, to make sure that you follow a balanced diet during the process. This is especially important for children, as excluding particular foods could lead to malnutrition and stunted growth.

Further information

Other methods of allergy and food intolerance testing are widely advertised – such as pulse-testing and applied kinesiology – but they haven't been proven to be reliable and are therefore best avoided. It's preferable to see your GP, or a qualified dietician. Your GP can access a directory produced by the British Society of Allergy and Clinical Immunology (BSACI), which lists specialist NHS Allergy Clinics in the UK, and may refer you to one if your test results warrant it. You can view this list yourself on the BSACI website – details are in the Directory at the end of the book; however, your GP needs to refer you to a clinic.

The Royal College of Pathologists offers a guide entitled *Allergy and Allergy Tests*, aimed at patients and relatives. Copies are available to download on their website, details of which can be found in the Directory at the end of the book.

Finally, lack of sleep can increase stress levels and exacerbate eczema. Certain foods and drinks may help to promote sleep. For more information on how to sleep better see Chapter 4 – Eczema and Emotions.

19. Sleep well with the right bedtime foods and drink

Eczema symptoms such as itching can disrupt your sleep and a lack of sleep can lead to you feeling stressed, which can exacerbate eczema. Apart from ensuring that you avoid your eczema triggers at bedtime – such as dust mites and an overheated room – and apply appropriate treatments, the following steps could help to improve the quality of your sleep.

Tryptophan-rich foods

Choose foods rich in tryptophan, an amino acid your body uses to produce serotonin – a substance which the brain converts into the 'sleep hormone' melatonin at night. Melatonin regulates sleep and is produced by the pineal gland in the brain, in response to darkness. Tryptophan-rich foods include bananas, chicken, turkey, dates, rice, oats, wholegrain breads and cereals. Ensure you're neither too hungry nor too full when you go to bed, as both can cause wakefulness.

Nature's tranquillisers

Calcium and magnesium have been dubbed 'nature's tranquilisers'. Both minerals soothe the nerves and relax the muscles, helping to promote restful sleep and avoid night cramps. Dairy products such as milk and cheese are good sources of calcium and also tryptophan – that's why a hot milky drink is an ideal night cap. Magnesium-rich foods include seafood, nuts, seeds, wholegrains and cooked green leafy vegetables. So an evening meal of chicken or turkey with brown rice or wholewheat pasta and cooked greens, followed by yogurt or cheese, would be conducive to sleep.

Avoid caffeine after 2 p.m.

Try not to drink coffee or cola after 2 p.m. as the stimulant effects of the caffeine they contain can last for hours. Whilst tea contains around half as much caffeine – around 50 mg per cup – it's best to avoid it near bedtime if you have sleep problems. Alternatively, try drinking rooibos tea, which is caffeine free, relaxing chamomile tea or decaffeinated coffee.

Drink alcohol in moderation

Drinking more than the recommended two units daily for women and three for men may relax you initially and help you fall asleep more quickly, but it has a stimulant effect, causing you to wake more often during the night. It's also a diuretic, making nocturnal trips to the toilet more likely. Some studies have suggested that drinking red wines such as Cabernet Sauvignon, Merlot or Chianti at bedtime promotes sleep because the grape skins they contain are rich in melatonin.

Chapter 4

Eczema and Emotions

This chapter looks at how emotions and stress can be linked to eczema flare-ups and how eczema symptoms can have an emotional impact, leading to a vicious circle of physical and emotional symptoms. Stress management and relaxation techniques are suggested to help prevent flare-ups and relieve tension during attacks. It also examines how support from fellow sufferers can help.

It's generally accepted that stress can contribute to eczema flare-ups in some individuals and some research suggests that emotions such as anger can play a part. For example, people with a 'type A' personality – tense, driven, aggressive, competitive and quick to anger – have been shown to be more likely to develop heart disease. A survey of 40 patients with long-standing atopic eczema at the Royal Melbourne Hospital in 1990 concluded they had high levels of anxiety, as well as problems in dealing with anger and hostility. A study in 1993 linked anxiety and feeling ineffective at handling anger to atopic eczema. Another study in 2001 suggested that stress worsened skin conditions such as eczema. Research in 2006 in Tokyo linked anxiety and depression to eczema flare-ups in predisposed individuals.

Equally, eczema can affect emotional well-being. In 2004, ISOLATE (International Study Of Life with Atopic Eczema) revealed that more than half of the 2,002 eczema sufferers who took part experienced bouts of depression and loss of self-confidence, as well as tension and difficulty relaxing during flare-ups. Respondents also reported that they felt embarrassment, anger and frustration because of their condition and many felt that their GPs failed to recognise the emotional impact of their eczema.

Skin and psyche

In order to understand how your mind can affect your skin, consider the links between the two. So that it can perceive and react to the surrounding environment, your skin contains numerous nerve endings, which link directly to your brain. So, for example, if one of your hands comes into contact with boiling water, or a sharp object, your brain responds by instructing you to remove it from the source of discomfort. In other words, your skin and your nervous system are intimately linked. Think of how your skin breaks out in a sweat in reaction to fear, how it can turn pale with shock, or red with embarrassment. The commonly used phrase 'thick skinned' is used to describe someone who is insensitive and hints of a connection between your skin and your emotions.

Dealing with feelings

American psychologist Ted Grossbart believes that it's not our emotions or feelings themselves that can cause skin problems, but rather how we deal with them. Grossbart explains that many of us bury our emotions in an attempt to protect ourselves from them. He asserts that if we don't allow ourselves to 'feel our feelings', we're more likely to develop physical symptoms, suggesting that eczema can be the result of suppressed emotions.

Grossbart claims he's had a lot of success in treating eczema sufferers using psychological techniques such as hypnosis, relaxation, visualisation and psychotherapy. A safe, simple self-hypnosis technique which incorporates relaxation and visualisation is outlined in Chapter 6 – DIY Complementary Therapies.

Let it all out!

If you tend to bottle up feelings, find ways to let your emotions out. Ideally, talk your feelings over with someone you can trust. If that isn't possible, try writing your feelings down on paper. If you're angry, try to identify what, or who, you feel angry about. Decide whether you can do anything about the situation. Can you avoid it happening again? Can you discuss your feelings with the person who has angered you? Often, the act of acknowledging our feelings can help to make us feel better.

If you're feeling sad and feel like crying, do so – it can provide social and psychological benefits. Crying in public can signal to others that we're unhappy and need emotional support and comfort. Crying in private is also beneficial, because when we cry we release stress hormones in our tears, suggesting it's the body's way of flushing out excess stress hormones – a kind of emotional safety valve.

Julie Graham's story

The experience of TV actress Julie Graham, who starred in the TV dramas *At Home with the Braithwaites* and *William and Mary*, lends weight to Dr Grossbart's theory. She suffered from facial eczema, which didn't respond to conventional treatments such as coal tar ointment and cortisone cream, for three years. In despair, she consulted a homeopath who suggested that her condition was linked to her mother's death three years earlier and the fact that she hadn't allowed herself to grieve properly. Once she realised that she had been bottling up her feelings, Julie started opening up to her friends and acknowledged her anger at the loss of her mother. She claims her eczema disappeared and hasn't returned – she believes her eczema was a symptom of the fact that she previously hadn't dealt with how she felt about her mother's death.

What is stress?

In a nutshell, stress is the way the mind and body respond to situations and pressures that leave us feeling inadequate or unable to cope. One person may cope well in a situation that another might find stressful. It's all down to the individual's perception of it and their ability to deal with it.

The brain reacts to stress by preparing the body to either stay put and face the perceived threat, or to escape from it. It does this by releasing hormones – chemical messengers – including adrenaline, noradrenaline and cortisol, into the bloodstream. These speed up the heart rate and breathing patterns and may induce sweating. Glucose and fatty acid levels in the blood rise to provide a burst of energy to deal with the threat. This is called the 'fight or flight' response.

These days the incidents that induce the stress response, e.g. pressure at work or financial problems, are on-going and unlikely to necessitate or be alleviated by either of these abrupt reactions, which means that stress hormone levels remain high. Over a prolonged period of time these chemicals can have a detrimental effect on health, leading to an increased risk of major health problems such as coronary heart disease as well as psychosomatic disorders (physical conditions caused or made worse by mental factors) such as eczema. So it's important to find ways to reduce and manage stress. Anxiety is part of this 'fight or flight' response to stress. Though it's a normal reaction to stressful situations, it can cause problems when it becomes part of the normal mindset.

The stress factor

It's quite widely accepted that stress can exacerbate atopic eczema. David Nicolson, a spokesperson for the Institute for Optimum Nutrition, said recently, 'The latest evidence suggests that eczema's connected with a depressed or overloaded immune system, as well as food intolerances. But one of the major trigger factors is stress.'

It's thought that stress hormones suppress the immune system, which can lead to an eczema flare-up in pre-disposed people. Also, research suggests that stress disrupts the production of sebum, thus lowering the efficiency of the skin barrier.

When stress triggers eczema...

Actress Claire Sweeney found that the stress of landing a role in the Channel 4 soap *Brookside* led to an eczema flare-up which covered her whole body.

Nadia Sawalha, former *EastEnders* actress and currently a TV presenter, had a similar experience when she suffered from severe eczema on her hands following her return to work shortly after the birth of her daughter.

Some experts have suggested that stress doesn't actually cause the eczema, but that some individuals scratch when they're stressed, which brings on an eczema attack. From a personal point of view, I don't believe this is the case. When my eczema used to flare-up on my eyelids and neck, I hadn't scratched these areas beforehand – the red angry patches of skin appeared first, then they started to itch and *then* I began to scratch!

If you feel that stress is a factor in your flare-ups you may benefit from finding ways to reduce your stress levels.

20. Identify your stress triggers

The stressful personality

As well as identifying external factors that make you feel stressed, consider whether some aspects of your personality are also to blame. Are you a perfectionist, who is never satisfied with your achievements and lifestyle? Constantly feeling that who you are and what you have aren't good enough can lead to unrealistic expectations, discontent and unnecessary stress. In his best-selling book, *Don't Sweat the Small Stuff*, Dr Richard Carlson urges us to remind ourselves that 'life is okay the way it is, right now'. Adopting this mindset immediately takes the pressure off and induces calm.

Workaholism is another stressor that's often linked to perfectionism – a 'perfect' home and lifestyle have to be paid for. And whilst working hard for the things you want in life is admirable, some people work such long hours they don't have time to enjoy what they have. If you're constantly driven to get everything done, believing that once everything on your 'to do list' is completed you'll be calm and relaxed, think again! What usually happens is that new 'to do' tasks appear, so your 'in basket' is never empty. Dr Carlson says he controls his obsession with completing his 'to do lists' by reminding himself that 'the purpose of life *isn't* to get it all done but to enjoy each step along the way'. He also advises, 'Remind yourself that when you die, your 'in basket' won't be empty.'

Perfectionism can also lead to the need to control – you convince yourself that no one else can meet your high standards, so you opt to do everything yourself. Insisting on doing everything yourself – whether at home or at work – inevitably leads to physical and mental overload. The solution is to accept that you can't know and do everything yourself and that it is beneficial to listen to other people's ideas and opinions and to delegate.

Keep a stress diary

For a couple of weeks, make a note of situations, times, places and people that make you feel stressed. Once you've identified your stressors you can then find ways to avoid or at least minimise them.

---

21. Just say 'no'

'No' is a little word that can reduce your stress levels dramatically. If you feel overburdened with chores and your stress levels are rising as a result, try saying 'no' to the non-essential tasks you don't have time for or simply don't want to do. If you find 'no' difficult to say, then perhaps you need to develop your assertiveness skills.

22. Be assertive

If you regularly find yourself giving in to others and not expressing how you feel to avoid hurting or upsetting them or to gain their approval, or if you regularly allow others to manipulate you into doing things you don't want to do, you could benefit from becoming more assertive. Being assertive means you can say what you want, feel and need, calmly and confidently, without being aggressive or hurting others. Use the following techniques to develop your self-assertiveness skills so that you can take control of your life and do things because *you* want to, rather than simply to please other people.

- Demonstrate ownership of your thoughts, feelings and behaviour by using 'I' rather than 'we', 'you', or 'it'. So rather than 'You make me angry' state 'I feel angry when you…'

- When you have a choice of whether to do something or not, say 'won't' rather than 'can't' to show you've made an active decision.

- Use 'choose to' instead of 'have to' and 'could' rather than 'should' to demonstrate that you have a choice whether or not to do something.

- When you feel your needs aren't being listened to, state what you want calmly and clearly, repeating it until the other person shows they've taken on board what you've said.

☐ When making a request, decide exactly what you want and what you're prepared to settle for. Use positive, assertive words, as outlined above.

☐ When refusing a request, speak firmly but calmly, giving the reason why, without apologising. Repeat if necessary.

☐ When you disagree with someone, say so using the word 'I'. State why you disagree, but accept the other person's right to have a different point of view.

23. Accept what you can't change

The serenity prayer tells us to accept the things we cannot change, have the courage to change the things we can, and the wisdom to know the difference. This isn't suggesting that you should just give up and accept that you can't change anything in your life, but rather that you should avoid wasting precious time and energy worrying about things over which you have no control, so that you can channel your efforts where they are of more benefit to you. Adopting such an attitude towards life can reduce stress levels substantially.

24. Change your perception

Changing your perception of situations can reduce feelings of stress. When something bad happens, instead of thinking about how bad the situation is, look for something positive about it if you can. Try to find solutions to your problems, or see them as an opportunity to grow. For example, being made redundant can seem like a terrible event, but if you view it as an opportunity to retrain and start a new career doing something you've always wanted to do it can become a catalyst for positive change.

25. Manage your time

If you regularly feel under pressure and stressed due to lack of time, try reviewing how you use it. Keep a diary for a few days to see how you spend your time and then identify which activities you can cut out, or reduce, to make time for the things that are most important to you. If you commute, try to use the time positively rather than just gazing out of the window. For example, read a book, schedule your activities for the week, or listen to your favourite music – a proven stress-reliever.

26. Eat a de-stress diet

What you eat also affects your mood and can heighten, or lower, the stress response. Chapter 3 looked at how a balanced diet is essential for healthy skin. Eating well also enables the body to deal with stress more efficiently by providing the essential fatty acids, B vitamins, calcium and magnesium that are needed for a healthy nervous system. A diet that includes plenty of wholegrains and little refined carbohydrate helps to maintain a steady blood sugar level by slowing down the rate at which glucose is absorbed, enabling the mind and body to function more efficiently, without stressful peaks and troughs in energy and mood.

Caffeine raises stress hormone levels, so a moderate daily intake of no more than 300 mg is advised. This is roughly the equivalent of three cups of brewed (or four cups of instant, coffee), six cups of tea and seven cans of cola.

Avoid resorting to alcohol to help you deal with stress. Drinking more than the recommended daily amounts (three to four units for men and two to three units for women) can increase stress by exacerbating depression and anxiety and disrupting sleep.

27. Get moving

Regular exercise is a great antidote to stress, because it enables the body to use up excess stress hormones. Their original purpose was to provide the extra energy needed to run away from our aggressors, or to stay put and fight – but in the absence of physical threats they build up in the body. It also triggers the release of endorphins, which improve mood and increase feelings of well-being.

28. Get back to nature

Get back to nature to help you relax and reduce your stress levels. Activities like going for a walk in the park, sitting in the garden or watching the sea have been shown to reduce heart rate, blood pressure and muscle tension. Experts believe that the higher levels of negative ions near areas with running water, trees and mountains may be partly responsible. Others claim it's due to 'biophilia' – the theory that we all have a natural affinity with nature and that our 'disconnection' from nature is the cause of mental health problems. Studies in the Netherlands and Japan show that people living in or near green areas enjoy a longer life and better health than those who live in urban environments.

29. Laugh more

Laughter is a great stress reliever. It seems that a good belly-laugh can reduce the stress hormones cortisol and adrenaline, and increase mood-boosting serotonin levels. People who see the funny side of life therefore have a reduced risk of the health problems associated with stress. So make time to watch your favourite comedies and be around people who make you laugh!

Have a hug!

Studies suggest that having a regular hug reduces stress hormones in the bloodstream and lowers blood pressure.

30. Breathe deep

When we're stressed our breathing tends to become shallow, or we hold our breath without realising it.

Slow, deep breathing has been shown to reduce the heart rate, relax muscles and release tension. So next time you're feeling stressed, try taking control of your breathing. Inhale slowly through your nostrils to a count of five, allowing your tummy to expand, hold for a count of five and then breathe out slowly through your nose to a count of five, whilst slowly flattening your stomach. Repeat up to ten times.

31. Focus on the here and now

Mindfulness, stemming from Buddhism, has been shown to reduce stress levels. It involves living in the present rather than worrying about the past or future. It's based on the idea that we can't change our past, or predict our future, but we can influence what's happening right now. By focussing fully on the present, you can carry out tasks to the best of your ability and make the most of each moment, whereas worrying about the past and future can hamper your performance and increase your stress levels unnecessarily.

32. Meditate

Meditation is a technique which, if practised regularly, has been shown to lower stress hormone levels, aid relaxation and soothe away anxiety.

Here's a simple meditation:

Whilst sitting comfortably, close your eyes. Breathe in through your nose deeply and slowly, inflating your stomach. Breathe out slowly and deeply through your mouth, deflating your stomach. As you continue to breathe in and out deeply, choose a word that suggests calmness, e.g. 'calm', 'peace', 'harmony' or just 'relax'. Repeat the word over and over in your mind, whilst visualising a place or an object that suggests calmness to you, for example, a flowing river or a flickering candle. Engage your other senses – imagine the sound of the water trickling by, feel the heat of the candle. Each time your mind wanders, acknowledge it, then re-focus on your chosen image and word.

To learn more go to www.t-m.org.uk.

33. Find social support

Research in 2003 at a hospital in Brazil suggested that joining a support group can be beneficial for eczema sufferers. Making contact with people who share the same condition can help beat the isolation and embarrassment many eczema sufferers feel. The following organisations offer the opportunity to do just that – further information and contact details are listed in the Directory at the end of the book:

- The National Eczema Society was formed in 1975 when a newspaper article showed there was a need for an information and support service for people with eczema and their carers. The society now provides a network of local contacts and support.

- Talk Eczema is a UK website set up by eczema sufferer Deborah Mason. The site offers a Message Board where you can read and post messages to other eczema sufferers. There's also a Find a Friend section which enables you to contact people with similar symptoms and interests.

- The Eczema Mailing List is an automated mailing list which offers eczema sufferers the opportunity to share their experiences with fellow sufferers.

- Eczema Voice, a UK website set up for people with eczema, offers a discussion board where you can read and leave messages.

34. Sleep well

Too little sleep has been shown to increase stress hormone levels in the bloodstream and can quickly have an effect on your skin, exacerbating eczema symptoms. Added to that, the itching eczema causes can disrupt sleep – leading to a seemingly never-ending cycle of poor sleep patterns, feeling stressed and worsening eczema. Clearly, the first step is to take steps to deal with the itch (see Chapter 2 – Skin Deep) – getting a good night's sleep is hard if your skin is constantly itching. Next, try the following tips to improve your chances of getting an adequate amount of good quality sleep, to reduce your stress levels and encourage your skin to heal itself.

Get outdoors during the day. Exposure to sunlight stops the production of melatonin – the brain chemical that induces sleep, making it easier for your body to produce it at night, so that you drop off more easily and sleep more soundly.

Being active can help you sleep more soundly, because it increases your body temperature and metabolism, which then fall a few hours later, promoting sleep. To benefit, don't exercise later than early evening. Being inactive all day can lead to restlessness and sleep difficulties.

Ensure your bedroom is cool and dark. Your brain tries to reduce your body temperature at night to slow down your metabolism. This is why an overly warm room can delay sleep. Being too hot may also make any itching worse. So to promote sleep aim for a temperature of around 16 °C. Darkness stimulates the body to produce melatonin. Use dark, heavy curtains, or line your current ones with blackout cloth. Alternatively, invest in some blackout blinds.

Avoid keeping a TV or computer in your bedroom. Watching TV or using a computer last thing at night may over-stimulate your brain, making it more difficult for you to unwind and drop off to sleep. The bright lights on TV and computer screens may also hinder the production of melatonin.

Soak in a warm bath at bedtime. The warmth raises your body temperature slightly. It then drops, encouraging sleep. Try adding a few drops of lavender or chamomile essential oils for their soothing, relaxing and calming properties.

Following a regular bedtime routine can promote sleep, as the brain learns to link dropping off with a particular sequence of events. For example, you might take a bath at the same time each night, before reading in bed with a milky drink. Taking time to relax before bed will help you to wind down and fall asleep more easily.

If mulling over problems or a busy schedule the next day prevents you falling asleep, try writing down your concerns or an action plan for the day before you go to bed.

Certain foods and drinks may help to boost the production of the sleep hormone melatonin and others can help you to relax (see Chapter 3 – Inside Out).

Chapter 5

Home Front

Your home can harbour many potential eczema triggers – house dust mites, chemical cleaners, air fresheners and pet hair, to name but a few. This chapter suggests changes you can make to your home environment and how you maintain it to help you reduce your exposure to these triggers and manage your symptoms. I believe that household cleaning products containing harmful chemicals are unnecessary when excellent results can be achieved using basic ingredients like white vinegar, lemon juice and bicarbonate of soda.

35. Control dust mites

House dust mites live on the human dead skin cells found in household dust. Some experts believe that the waste matter from house dust mites can be an eczema trigger for some people. Studies have suggested that cutting the number of dust mites in your home can reduce eczema symptoms, but others report no effect. It seems that mainly children show improvement when dust mites are controlled.

Come clean

Clean rooms thoroughly each week. Wipe floors, furniture, window sills and frames and even door tops with a damp cloth to remove dust.

Go carpet-free

Carpet fibres can harbour dust and are therefore an ideal home for dust mites, making hard floors a better alternative; the current trend for wooden and tiled floors is beneficial for eczema sufferers, because dust and dirt are more visible and they're easier to keep clean.

Curtain call

Use blinds rather than curtains as they're easier to keep dust free. However, avoid venetian blinds – they tend to gather dust and are more difficult to clean. Roman blinds, roller blinds, pleated and vertical blinds are relatively easy to keep dust free – try using the brush attachment on your vacuum cleaner.

Cuddly toy chiller

Children's cuddly toys are an ideal home for dust mites. One way of killing the dust mites is to put soft toys in the freezer. Dust mites die at temperatures below 20 °C. Wash afterwards to remove droppings.

Bedding blitz

The dust mite's favourite haunt is in your bedding. To reduce numbers, pull back the bedclothes every morning and allow the bed to air for at least an hour – preferably with the window open. Wash sheets, duvet covers and pillowcases once a week at 60 °C. Vacuum the mattress before replacing the bedding. Wash duvets and pillows as often as possible. Those made from synthetic fibres are easier to wash than those with feathers. Where possible, hang washing outside to dry. You can also buy mite-resistant pillows and duvets and mite-resistant covers for your mattress and duvet – see the Useful Products section for further details.

Keep rooms airy

Mites like warm, damp conditions. To keep mites at bay, ensure your home's humidity level stays between 45 and 55 per cent. If you suspect the atmosphere in your home is too damp or too dry, use a hygrometer, a device that measures humidity, to check the amount of moisture in the air. Opening your windows every day will help to reduce humidity. Bowls of water around the house will increase it. Or you can use dehumidifiers or humidifiers to achieve the ideal humidity level. For details of where you can buy a compact hygrometer, see the Useful Products section.

36. Control temperature

Extreme heat or cold can aggravate some types of eczema, including atopic, so it's important to dress appropriately – preferably in cotton, with extra layers in winter. Keep your house as cool as possible in the summer and don't have the thermostat set too high in the winter. Keep your bedroom fairly cool – a temperature of below 16 °C (61 °F) will reduce the risk of sweating, which can exacerbate itching, and aid restful sleep. Sudden changes in temperature can trigger itching, so wrap up well before going outside in cold weather.

37. Solve your pet problems

If you discover that pet hair, or dander, is a trigger for your eczema, you obviously need to avoid contact with them. If you're a pet owner this can be very difficult! There are products available that are aimed at removing allergens from pets' coats. These usually take the form of lotions or shampoos that are rubbed into the fur and then wiped, or rinsed off, taking the allergens with them.

The manufacturers of one such product, Petal Cleanse, a product designed to ease the problem, claim that it's not just hair and dander that are to blame, but also saliva, urine and allergens. The manufacturer states that in clinical trials 90 per cent of people with pet allergies benefited from using their product to remove these irritants from their pets' coats. For more details see the Useful Products section.

38. Glove up

Shield the skin on your hands by wearing protective gloves. Use rubber ones when washing up, using cleaning products or for jobs involving putting your hands in water. Wear cotton gloves underneath if you have an allergy to latex. Wear gardening gloves when gardening, as some plants can cause skin irritation. These include primulas, tulips, chrysanthemums and ivy. Put gloves on when you go outdoors in cold weather. Cold air, windy conditions and low humidity can dry out the skin on your hands and exacerbate your eczema. Companies such as The Healthy House Ltd and Allergy Best Buys sell pure cotton gloves. For further details see the Useful Products section.

39. Clean naturally

In the introduction we discussed how chemical-based household cleaners are another potential hazard in your home that can trigger eczema symptoms. In a recent study by the World Wildlife Fund involving 47 volunteers, between 13 and 54 out of 101 man-made chemicals were detected in individual volunteers' bodies. Many of these were found to have come from household cleaning products and were identified as harmful. Instead of using products laden with chemicals, opt for eco-friendly cleaners based on natural ingredients such as lemon or vinegar – for further details go to the Useful Products Section. Alternatively, you can make your own using items from your kitchen cupboard, such as vinegar, lemons, salt and bicarbonate of soda.

Bleach substitute

Borax (a natural mineral salt containing boron) can be used as a gentler alternative to bleach. To remove stains on white cotton or linen, apply directly then rinse. Soak coloured fabrics in a weak solution of borax – made by adding 20 g (one tablespoon) to 500 ml (one pint) of water – for no longer than 15 minutes. For an all-purpose household cleaner and disinfectant, mix one teaspoon of borax with two tablespoons of white vinegar and one litre of hot water.

Soda solution

Bicarbonate of soda is cheap and highly versatile. Mixed with water, it forms an alkaline solution that helps dissolve dirt and grease and neutralise smells. It can be used on carpets to remove stains. To clean a smelly drain, sprinkle one cupful of bicarbonate of soda into it, then slowly pour one cup of white vinegar down. The resulting foam degreases and deodorises. Sprinkled on a damp cloth, it acts as a mild abrasive that removes marks from surfaces without scratching. Use it in this way on plastic, porcelain, glass, tiles and stainless steel. Use it in the bathroom to scour the bath and washbasin and in the kitchen to clean your fridge, freezer, microwave, cooker top and oven. Fill a small container with bicarbonate and leave in the fridge to absorb odours. Stir it now and again and replace every three months. To clean and freshen your dishwasher add one cup of bicarbonate and run it on the rinse cycle whilst empty. For tough stains, mix with a little water to make a paste, apply and leave for a few minutes, before rinsing off. Silver and jewellery emerge clean and shiny when cleaned in this way.

Lemon fresh

Lemons contain citric acid, which makes them great natural cleaners, with bleaching, antiseptic, antibacterial and degreasing qualities. Use half a lemon to clean the bath and washbasin. Rubbing it on and around the taps will remove limescale and leave them gleaming – especially if you buff them afterwards with a dry cloth. To clean copper and brass, dip half a lemon into salt and rub. Rinse well straight away to prevent discolouration. Lemon is also a natural bleach – to brighten clothing and bed linen, soak them in a bucket of water to which you've added the juice of a lemon and leave overnight before washing as normal. Lemon also deodorises. To clean your microwave and remove food smells, place a couple of slices of lemon into a microwaveable bowl containing water. Microwave for a couple of minutes, then wipe using kitchen roll or a clean cloth. To keep your fridge fresh, place a couple of slices of lemon inside.

Natural polish

Olive oil is a good natural substitute for commercial furniture polish. Simply mix a cup of ordinary olive oil – it doesn't need to be extra-virgin – with the juice of one lemon and pour it into a spray bottle. To polish wooden surfaces, spray a little on to the surface and rub. The lemon juice cuts through the dirt, whilst the olive oil shines and protects the wood. Use a dry cloth to remove the excess oil and buff to a shine. Use sparingly, as excessive amounts of oil could leave the surface feeling tacky. Olive oil is also good for getting rid of fingerprints on stainless steel surfaces and cooking utensils. Simply sprinkle a little on some kitchen roll and buff.

Value vinegar

Vinegar is a dilute solution of acetic acid that cuts through grease, deodorises and is mildly disinfectant. White vinegar is the best type to use around your home, as it doesn't have a strong smell. Mix equal amounts of white vinegar and water in a spray bottle and use as a general cleaner. It's especially good on tiles and kitchen worktops. For a fresh fragrance add a few drops of lemongrass, bergamot or geranium essential oils. For difficult stains, use warm water. Cover the stain and leave for ten minutes before wiping off. White vinegar also makes a great window cleaner – use half a cup in a litre of warm water. Simply spray onto your window and then remove and buff with crumpled newspapers to avoid streaking.

Vinegar is a good de-scaler, as it can dissolve lime deposits. To clean a showerhead, simply remove it and soak in undiluted vinegar. To remove limescale from your kettle, fill it up with vinegar and leave overnight. Pour the liquid out the next day and rinse well before using. To de-scale taps, soak a few paper towels in white vinegar. Wrap them around the taps and then cover them with plastic bags held in place with elastic bands. Leave for a few hours before rinsing and buffing to a shine with a dry cloth.

Ketchup cleaner

If you've run out of vinegar, tomato ketchup makes a good, if slightly messy, substitute as it contains acetic acid. It's especially recommended for cleaning copper and brass.

Minty air freshener

Instead of using commercial air fresheners to remove bad smells, try making your own. Fill a spray bottle with white vinegar and add about twenty drops of peppermint essential oil. Shake well before spraying. Avoid spraying near your eyes, as vinegar can irritate them.

Natural disinfectant

Australian tea-tree oil – *Melaleuca alternifolia* – is an excellent disinfectant and fungicide. For a general-purpose disinfectant solution mix 10 ml (two teaspoons) of tea-tree oil with two cups of water. To remove and reduce mould and mildew growth use the solution in a spray bottle and squirt on the affected areas. Leave for a few minutes and then rinse with warm, soapy water. To keep shower curtains mildew free and to remove strong mildewy smells from fabrics, add a few drops of tea tree-oil to your usual washing powder.

Ready-made non-allergenic natural cleaning products

If you'd prefer to buy ready made non-allergenic natural cleaning products, Ecover – a range of cleaning products manufactured using plant-based ingredients – is available at most supermarkets. Many supermarkets now produce their own brand plant-based ranges.

40. Use non-biological washing powders

Eczema sufferers have traditionally been advised to avoid biological washing powders and choose non-biological powders instead. A recent review of the evidence concluded that detergents containing enzymes were no harsher on the skin than non-biological alternatives. However, Lyndsey McManus, spokesperson for the charity Allergy UK, commented that many people find non-bio powders kinder to their skin. It's really a case of seeing what works best for you. If you feel that the enzymes or perhaps the perfumes in biological powders do worsen your symptoms, then you may be better off avoiding them. Try removing stubborn stains by mixing salt with white vinegar to form a paste and rubbing in before washing. You can also buy laundry balls to use instead of detergents in the washer. These leave no residue on clothes. Some contain mineral salts, which ionise the water. See the Useful Products section for further details. Wash your clothes on a double rinse cycle to remove all traces of soap powder or fabric softener.

41. Use water softeners

A study in Nottingham showed that eczema is more prevalent in schoolchildren living in hard water areas. This may be because hard water contains calcium and magnesium salts that may irritate the skin, or it could be because people living in hard water areas tend to use more soaps and detergents, which exacerbate symptoms. Water softeners may improve symptoms, but there's no conclusive evidence that this is the case. They soften water by removing calcium and magnesium salts. If you want to try a water softener for yourself make sure you buy from a reputable company. Only ion exchange water softeners will completely eradicate hardness. For more information visit The National Eczema Society's website – the details are in the Directory.

Natural ingredients

A company called The Soap Kitchen sells many of the ingredients I've mentioned. The contact details can be found in the Useful Products section.

Chapter 6

DIY Complementary Therapies

Complementary therapies seek to treat the whole person rather than simply the symptoms. The emphasis is on supporting the body, to enable it to heal itself. Whilst it's unlikely any complementary treatment will 'cure' your eczema, some may help you to feel less stressed and improve your well-being – which may in turn reduce the number of flare-ups you have.

In this chapter I've included a brief overview and evaluation of the usefulness of alternative approaches, such as naturopathy and reflexology. I've also suggested which aspects you could adopt within your own self-help programme, such as a wholefood diet and simple reflexology techniques.

42. Use essential oils

Essential oils are extracted by various means from the petals, leaves, stalk, roots, seeds, nuts and even the bark of plants. Aromatherapy is based on the theory that when scents released from essential oils are inhaled, they affect the hypothalamus. This is the part of the brain that governs the glands and hormones, altering mood and lowering stress. When used in massage, baths and compresses, the oils are also absorbed through the bloodstream and transported to the organs and glands, which benefit from their healing effects. A couple of studies have suggested that essential oils such as neroli, valerian and lavender can aid relaxation and induce calm. Since eczema is often linked to emotional stress, aromatherapy may be worth trying, both as a preventative measure and during a flare-up. Oils may also have anti-inflammatory, moisturising or healing properties.

Patricia Davis, author of *Aromatherapy: An A-Z*, recommends blending essential oils with an aqueous cream or non-perfumed lotion, as carrier oils such as almond or wheatgerm can sometimes exacerbate skin conditions. With most essential oils, use a 1 per cent dilution – this equates to one drop per teaspoon of aqueous cream or lotion. Never apply aromatherapy oils to broken skin.

Chamomile

Chamomile has been used medicinally for thousands of years. It is believed to soothe and calm both the mind and skin and is thus of special benefit since emotional stress is often involved in an eczema flare-up. If large areas of skin are affected, add about six drops of chamomile essential oil, or even a couple of chamomile teabags, to your bath.

Local application of chamomile has been shown to be moderately effective in the treatment of eczema. In a double-blind trial it was found to be around 60 per cent as effective as 0.25 per cent hydrocortisone cream.

Lemon balm

If chamomile doesn't bring about an improvement, lemon balm is worth trying, since it has similar properties to chamomile. Lemon balm is quite a strong oil, so for best results mix one drop with two teaspoons of unperfumed lotion or aqueous cream.

Lavender
Lavender may also ease eczema. It has soothing, antiseptic and anti-inflammatory properties and also soothes and calms the emotions and boosts mood. So, like the previous two oils, it may help to relieve symptoms by tackling both the underlying cause and the actual condition.

Geranium
Geranium is recommended for dry eczema. It has healing, antiseptic properties and helps to balance the skin's natural oils – correcting excessive dryness. It also has antidepressant qualities, so it can help with any underlying psychological factors. To benefit, add six drops to the bath, or apply it directly to the affected area, diluted in unperfumed lotion or aqueous cream.

Patchouli
Patchouli oil is often recommended for its aphrodisiac qualities, but its anti-inflammatory and antiseptic properties mean it's useful for treating eczema – especially where the skin is dry or cracked.

43. Help yourself with homeopathy

Homeopathy literally means 'same suffering' and is based on the idea that 'like cures like' – substances that can cause symptoms in a well person can treat the same symptoms in a person who is ill. Symptoms like inflammation or fever are viewed as a sign that the body is trying to heal itself. The theory is that the homeopathic remedies stimulate this self-healing process and they work in a similar way to vaccines.

How homeopathy works

The substances used in homeopathic remedies come from plant, animal and mineral sources. These substances are made into a tincture, which is then diluted many times. Homeopaths claim that the more diluted a remedy is, the higher its potency and the lower its potential side effects. They believe in the 'memory of water', a theory suggesting that although molecules from substances have been diluted away, they've left behind an electromagnetic 'footprint' – rather like a recording on an audio tape – which has an effect on the body. Research suggests that the high dilutions of substances in homeopathic remedies reduce the risk of adverse effects.

These ideas are controversial and many GPs remain sceptical. Evidence to support homeopathy exists, but much of it is deemed inconclusive. For example, research published in 2005 reported improvements in symptoms and well-being among 70 per cent of patients receiving individualised homeopathy. The study involved 6,500 patients over a six-year period at the Bristol Homeopathic Hospital. Sixty-eight per cent of eczema sufferers under the age of 16 reported feeling 'better' or 'much better'. Critics of the studies argue that there was no comparison group and patients may have given a positive response because they felt that was what the researchers wanted to hear. That said, many people claim to have been helped by homeopathy, so it may well be worth trying.

There are two main types of remedies – whole person based and symptom based. A homeopath would prescribe a remedy aimed at you as a whole person, based on your personality as well as the symptoms you experience. The homeopathic view of eczema is that it's a disease linked to the metabolic system, whereby the skin is trying to offload toxins in the bloodstream. The easiest way to treat yourself is to select a remedy that most closely matches your particular eczema symptoms. Below are the remedies most often prescribed for eczema and the particular symptoms for which they're believed to treat.

Arsenicum Album
Suggested for dry, itchy skin that's made worse by cold temperatures.

Dulcamara
Recommended for weeping, crusted eczema that's exacerbated by damp conditions.

Graphites
Recommended where eczema is moist with oozing, itchy, cracked skin.

Lycopodium
Recommended for dry, scaly skin – with no infection.

Natrum mur.
For moist eczema without an itch, but with a burning, watery discharge.

Petroleum

For moist eczema with roughened, broken skin or crusting, brought on by stress and worse at night.

Rhus tox.

For red, burning, itchy eczema with scaly skin, which worsens in cold, damp weather but improves in the warmth.

Sulphur

Recommended if your eczema is dry, scaly and very itchy and especially if your symptoms worsen with scratching, warmth and bathing.

Calcerea carbonica

May bring relief to eczema accompanied by cracked and itching skin that's worse in cold and damp weather.

44. Try hypnotherapy

Trance-like states have been used for centuries by different cultures to encourage healing. The founder of modern hypnosis was Franz Anton Mesmer, whose method of treating patients was termed 'mesmerism'. Hypnotherapists encourage a state of mind that's similar to deep daydreaming and promotes deep relaxation and openness to suggestion.

The Royal College of Physicians Committee on Clinical Immunology and Allergy concluded in 1992 that hypnosis might have a small role to play in helping the asthmatic. Brain scans have shown that hypnotic suggestion can sometimes have an observable effect on the brains of some people. Studies suggest that as well as being relaxing – which in itself can be beneficial to eczema sufferers – hypnosis may boost immune function and that visualisation may improve skin rashes. One study showed that hypnotherapy and biofeedback – the use of monitoring equipment to measure and encourage relaxation – reduced skin damage and thickening. Another trial in 1995 suggested that hypnosis reduced itching, scratching and sleep problems in both children and adults.

Simple self-hypnosis

Most people can learn safe and simple self-hypnosis techniques. The following steps will take you through a basic self-hypnosis, which could aid relaxation and positive thinking and possibly help to ease eczema symptoms.

1. Lie or sit comfortably in a quiet place, where you're unlikely to be disturbed.

2. Focus on your breathing – breathe slowly and deeply.

3. Start counting backwards from 300. If your mind starts to drift away, simply start counting backwards again.

4. At the same time, start relaxing each part of your body. Allow the muscles in your face to relax, then those in your neck and shoulders, back, arms and legs and finally your feet.

5. Now repeat affirmations – positive statements about yourself – as though they're already true, e.g. 'I'm calm and relaxed in all situations' or 'My skin is smooth and healthy'.

6. When you're ready to come out of your trance start counting to ten, telling yourself 'When I reach five I'll start to awaken; when I reach ten I'll wake up, feeling calm and relaxed.'

45. Visualise healthy skin

Visualisation involves using your imagination to create a picture in your mind of the situation you want to achieve. It's claimed that the more senses you use in your visualisation the more effective it's likely to be. Using visualisation during self-hypnosis appears to improve its success and is called hypnotic imaging.

Follow the self-hypnosis techniques outlined above. As you make an affirmation, experience it in your subconscious, as though it's happening now, by conjuring up a scene in which you've already achieved your goal. For example, if your affirmation is 'My skin is clear and healthy', see, hear and feel it. Picture your skin glowing and healthy, hear your friends and family commenting on how good your skin looks and 'feel' its softness and smoothness.

46. Enjoy a massage

One study showed that massage for 20 minutes each day improved the symptoms of children with atopic eczema and reduced anxiety. Since anxiety has been shown to exacerbate eczema symptoms in some people, any improvement is likely to be due to the relaxing effects of massage.

Massage involves touch, which can ease away tensions. It seems to work by stimulating the release of endorphins – the body's own painkillers – plus serotonin, a brain chemical implicated in relaxation. It also decreases the level of stress hormones in the blood and improves blood circulation.

Mix your own massage oil by combining a few drops of your favourite aromatherapy oil (e.g. lavender, chamomile or ylang-ylang) into a carrier oil such as almond or grapeseed, or an unperfumed lotion or aqueous cream if the area to be massaged is affected by eczema. An easy way to benefit from massage is for you and a partner to massage each other's back, neck and shoulders, using the basic techniques outlined below:

Stroking/effleurage – slide both hands over the skin in rhythmic fanning or circular motions.

Kneading – using alternate hands, squeeze and release flesh between the fingers and thumbs, as though you're kneading dough.

Friction – using your thumbs, apply even pressure to static points, or make small circles on both sides of the spine.

Hacking – relax your hands then, using the sides, speedily and alternately give short, sharp taps all over.

Playing some relaxing music in the background can enhance the feelings of relaxation.

47. Turn to naturopathy

Naturopathy means 'nature cure' and is based on the philosophy that illness occurs when the body's natural equilibrium is upset by an unhealthy lifestyle. Naturopaths believe that factors such as an unhealthy diet, insufficient sleep, lack of fresh air, little exercise, emotional and physical stress and pollution cause a build-up of toxins, which can lead to a weakened immune system and susceptibility to bacteria, viruses and allergens. Symptoms such as eczema are seen as signs of the body attempting to heal itself and it's thought that, rather than suppressing such symptoms, the body's self-healing ability should be supported with a healthy lifestyle. A practitioner will try to find out why a person has become ill and then suggest lifestyle changes to restore balance and good health. Detoxification is central to naturopathy.

To promote efficient digestion and elimination of toxins, an eczema sufferer would initially be advised to follow a restricted diet based on fruit, vegetables and grains. Such a diet would probably be supplemented with herbs such as burdock to cleanse and tone the liver. Evidence suggests that a wholefood diet and naturopathic approaches to stress management and fitness, such as yoga and massage, can lead to improved health.

48. Try flower remedies

Flower essences have been used for their healing properties for thousands of years, but it was Dr Edward Bach, a Harley Street doctor, bacteriologist and homeopath, who developed their use in the UK in the twentieth century. In the 1930s he studied his patients and concluded that mental attitude played a vital role both in health and recovery from illness. He identified 38 basic negative states of mind and developed a plant- or flower-based remedy for each. By 1936 Bach was producing his remedies commercially. The remedies are believed to counteract stress and negative emotions such as despair, fear and uncertainty, but there's only anecdotal evidence as to their effectiveness. Today they're widely available in pharmacies in 10 and 20 ml phials that are convenient for carrying. The remedies are taken by diluting two drops in a glass of water, or they can be dropped directly onto the tongue. If you suspect that your emotions are implicated in your eczema, you may find that one of the following remedies help.

Impatiens
This remedy is recommended if your eczema makes you feel irritable and self-conscious.

Mimulus
Indicated for skin that's hypersensitive – especially if you think your eczema is linked to anxiety.

Agrimony
This flower essence is useful if you think your eczema might be linked to bottled-up feelings.

For further information to help you choose a suitable flower remedy and an online questionnaire that enables you to select a personalised blend, visit www.bachfloweressences.co.uk.

49. Find relief in reflexology

Reflexology is based on the theory that points on the feet, hands and face known as reflexes correspond to parts of the body, glands and organs. Stimulating these reflexes using the fingers and thumbs brings about physiological changes which encourage the mind and body to self-heal. Practitioners believe that imbalances in the body result in granular deposits in the relevant reflex, leading to tenderness. Corns, bunions and even hard skin are thought to indicate problems in the parts of the body their position is linked to. Whilst medical opinion is divided, evidence suggests that foot and hand massage can reduce stress.

Here are some techniques you can try for yourself; one is to reduce stress, since it's often implicated in eczema and the other to aid digestion, which may also be a factor. They involve working on your hands, as this is easier than treating your own feet.

To relieve stress: use the thumb of your right hand to apply pressure to the solar plexus reflex on your left hand. It's located about two-thirds of the way up, in line with the centre of your middle finger. Repeat on your right hand, using your left thumb.

To improve digestion: use the thumb of your left hand to apply pressure to the middle third of your right palm in a creeping movement, working from left to right for two minutes. Do the same with your left palm, using your right thumb and working from right to left.

50. Say 'yes' to yoga

Yoga may be beneficial for eczema sufferers because it's thought to relieve stress. It's a gentle form of exercise that helps to calm the mind and is less likely to cause sweating, which can irritate the skin during an eczema flare-up. The word 'yoga' comes from the Sanskrit word *yuj*, meaning union. Yogic postures and breathing exercises are designed to unite the body, mind and soul. Inverted postures, such as the shoulder stand, boost circulation and blood flow to the upper body, helping to increase alertness and improve the skin. Some sufferers find that yoga breathing helps them to relax and that it draws their attention away from their itchy skin.

Yogic breathing

If it is practical to do so, sit on a carpet or mat with your legs crossed or straight out in front of you, with your hands resting on your knees. However, this isn't essential – the most important thing is to ensure you're sitting comfortably, with your head, neck and spine aligned. Breathe in slowly through your nostrils, allowing first your stomach and then your ribcage to expand. Hold for a count of ten and then slowly exhale, flattening your stomach and releasing your ribcage.

Learn yoga

The best way to learn yoga is by attending classes run by a qualified teacher. To find one near you, go to the British Wheel of Yoga's website – www.bwy.org.uk. Or, if you'd prefer to teach yourself at home, visit www.abc-of-yoga.com – a site which shows you how to perform yoga poses (asanas) and offers information about yoga and the benefits of practising it. When practising yoga at home make sure you proceed gently and don't force your body into postures. Always stop if you feel any discomfort. Wear lightweight, loose clothing to allow you to move freely and no footwear, as yoga is best performed barefoot. Use a non-slip mat if the floor is slippery. Don't attempt inverted postures if you have a neck or back problem, or have high blood pressure, heart disease or circulatory problems. If in doubt, consult your GP first.

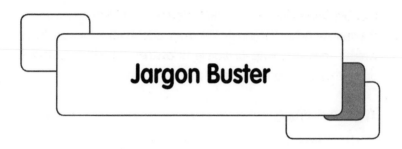

Jargon Buster

Acute – something that starts suddenly and is soon over. Eczema tends to be a long-lasting condition with acute flare-ups.

Allergens – substances that cause allergies, e.g. pollen, pet dander and foods such as peanuts.

Allergy – an extreme response by the immune system to a normally harmless substance – involves the production of a harmful antibody known as IgE.

Anaphylaxis – also known as anaphylactic shock. A severe, potentially fatal allergic reaction.

Antihistamine – a drug that blocks the effects of histamine.

Anti-inflammatory – a drug or other substance that counteracts inflammation.

Atopic – allergic.

Chronic – persistent, long-lasting.

Dermis – the thick, inner layer of your skin, beneath the epidermis.

Double-blind – a trial in which information which may influence the behaviour of the investigators or the participants (such as which participants have been given a placebo rather than an active treatment) is withheld.

Emollient – a moisturiser that helps to keep moisture in the skin.

Epidermis – the thin, outer layer of the skin.

Erythema – redness caused by acute inflammation.

Histamine – a substance released by the immune system in response to an allergen.

Inflammation – a response by the immune system, designed to protect the body from invasion by foreign substances. Symptoms include redness, heat, swelling and pain.

Integrative medicine – healing-oriented medicine that takes the whole person (body, mind and spirit) into account, including all aspects of lifestyle. It makes use of both conventional and alternative therapies.

Intolerance – hypersensitivity to a substance that doesn't involve the immune response and is therefore not a true allergy. Some people term it a 'hidden allergy'.

Lichenification – thickening of the skin, resulting from persistent scratching.

Psychosomatic – literally means 'mind and body'. Usually used to describe diseases thought to be made worse by states of mind such as stress and anxiety.

Pruritus – itching.

Sebum – an oily secretion that forms part of the skin barrier.

Sensitivity – a response by the immune system to a particular substance.

Steroids (corticosteroids) – drugs with anti-inflammatory properties, similar to the steroid hormones produced by the adrenal glands.

Urticaria – a rash resembling nettle rash, with itchy, fluid-filled lumps – a sign of an allergic response.

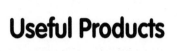

Useful Products

Below is a list of products and suppliers of products that may help to ease eczema symptoms. The author doesn't endorse or recommend any particular product and this list is by no means exhaustive – there is a vast range of products that may help with the prevention and treatment of eczema.

Allergenics

A range of skincare products for dry skin that are made from hypoallergenic ingredients such as aloe vera and borage oil and are fragrance, lanolin and preservative free. The main ingredient is soya bean phytosterols, which are thought to have a similar effect to cortisone.
Telephone: 01903 821 550
Website: www.allergenics.co.uk

Aloe Propolis Crème

Contains aloe vera gel and bee propolis, a natural antibiotic.
Website: www.aloeveraproductsonline.co.uk

Aloe Vera Gelly

A thick gel containing aloe vera.
Website: www.aloeveraproductsonline.co.uk

Aquaball Laundry Ball

Cleans clothes without detergent. It works by releasing ionised oxygen, which aids dirt removal.
Website: www.healthy-house.co.uk

Baby Salve

A natural rescue salve especially formulated for babies, but also suitable for people who may be prone to eczema, psoriasis and dermatitis. Contains organic hemp, calendula and lavender; is free from lanolin, petrochemicals and parabens.
Address: The Green People, Pondtail Farm, Coolham Road, West Grinstead, West Sussex, RH13 8LN
Telephone: 01403 740 350
Email: organic@greenpeople.co.uk
Website: www.greenpeople.co.uk

Bach Rescue Cream

A skin salve containing a blend of six Bach Flower Essences. Soothes and moisturises rough, dry skin to restore it to its natural good condition. Bach Rescue Cream is available in a 30 g tube.
Website: www.bachfloweressences.co.uk

Balneum

A range of products, including bath oils and creams, containing ingredients such as urea (which has moisturising properties), soya oil and lauromacrogols (which have an anaestheticising effect).
Website: www.chemistdirect.co.uk

Bionaire Compact Ultrasonic Humidifier

A compact 1.4 l cool mist humidifier treated with Microban Antimicrobial Product Protection.
Website: www.bionaireuk.co.uk

Cardiospermum Gel

A natural hypoallergenic gel containing cardiospermum plant extract, which is thought to have an anti-inflammatory effect, as well as Aloe Vera extract. The gel was tested by over 100 eczema sufferers before it was made available for purchase. The company also produces Dry Skin Eye Gel, which contains slightly less cardiospermum, to help with dry skin and eczema around the eyes.

Telephone: 0871 871 9975
Website: www.skinshop.co.uk

Compact Hygrometer

A low-priced hygrometer that measures both relative humidity and air temperature – suitable for domestic use. Available from Thermometers Direct.

Website: www.thermometersdirect.co.uk

Crystal Ball Bath Dechlorinator

A plastic ball containing a filter that transforms chlorine to harmless zinc chloride. It can be hung from a bath tap, or swished around the bath water a few times. Lasts for up to 12 months. The filter inside the ball can be replaced.

Website: www.pureandgentleskincare.com

DermaSalve

A range of moisturising creams which are free from all known common irritants. Products contain natural oils, grapeseed extract and aloe vera to moisturise and soothe, and the antioxidants vitamins C and E to improve skin condition. DermaSalve products are light and non-greasy, and the moisturising effect lasts for up to 12 hours. Products include infant and baby, body, face, hand, foot and heel creams and a laundry powder. Recommended by Dr Chris Steele from ITV's *This Morning*.

Website: www.PN4H.com

Derma Veen

A range of products that includes shampoo, moisturising lotion for hands, face and body, shower and bath oil and soap free wash. Products contain colloidal oatmeal to soothe itching, and sodium PCA to retain moisture in the skin.

Website: www.pureandgentle.com

Dust Mite Proof Bedding

The Healthy House Ltd offers a wide range of dust mite proof bedding and dust mite proof bedding covers.

Website: www.healthy-house.co.uk

E45 Cream

A non-greasy emollient that's been clinically proven to treat and soothe dry, itchy, flaky, rough or chapped skin. Other products in the range include bath oil, lotion, hand wash and dry scalp shampoo.

Website: www.e45.com

E45 Suncare

A range of sun protection products especially formulated for sensitive skins. Includes sun lotion and sun screen. Available in SPFs 15 and 30.

Website: www.e45.com

Ecoballs

Use these eco-friendly laundry balls instead of detergent, to avoid skin irritation. Each Ecoball contains mineral salts that produce ionised oxygen, which lifts the dirt. Each set of three of three Ecoballs lasts for up to 1,000 washes.

Website: www.ecozone.co.uk

Eczema Clothing Ltd

A company specialising in clothing made from 100 per cent organic cotton for those with eczema, allergies and sensitive skin. Also produces nightwear using 'natural silver soothe', a fabric containing natural silver to ease night-time itching and prevent secondary infection.

Telephone: 01772 331 815

Website: www.eczemaclothing.com

Epaderm

Developed by doctors at the Royal Victoria Infirmary, Newcastle-upon-Tyne, Epaderm is a pale yellow ointment containing emulsifying wax and yellow soft paraffin, liquid paraffin and no fragrances, colourings or additives. It provides a film barrier which aids moisture retention and can be used on the skin, in the bath, or as a skin cleanser.

Website: www.skincareworld.co.uk

Eucerin Dry Skin Relief Soothing Spray

A light, spray-on moisturiser recommended by Talk Eczema for the relief of dry, itchy skin. Contains cooling menthol, evening primrose oil to replenish the skin's natural oils and other ingredients which are clinically proven to reduce itching and moisturise the skin. Other Eucerin products include face, hand and foot creams containing urea, which increases moisture retention in the skin.

Website: www.echemist.co.uk

Gloves in a Bottle

A lotion designed to bond with the outer layer of skin to form a protective shield that works like an invisible pair of gloves. It prevents exposure to harmful irritants and allows the skin's natural barrier to be restored. It doesn't wash off – it comes off naturally with exfoliated skin cells – but it needs to be reapplied every four hours.

Recommended by many dermatologists for both atopic eczema and also irritant contact dermatitis on the hands.
Telephone: 0800 3894710
Website: www.allergybestbuys.co.uk

HC45 Hydrocortisone Cream
A low-dose hydrocortisone cream available from pharmacies without prescription.
Website: www.e45.com

The Healthy House Cotton Gloves
Suitable for eczema sufferers – especially those suffering from latex allergy. They come in two styles and in various adult's and children's sizes. The Healthy House Ltd is a UK based company offering a wide range of products for those who suffer from allergies and sensitivities, including eczema. Other products include natural creams to moisturise and improve skin condition, anti-allergy clothing, bedding, carpets and paint.
Address: The Old Co-op, Lower Street, Ruscombe, Stroud, Gloucestershire, GL6 6BU
Telephone: 0845 450 5950
Website: www.healthy-house.co.uk

Hypericum and Calendula Cream
An antiseptic and soothing cream, which contains organically produced sunflower oil, olive oil, St John's Wort extract and calendula extract. Available from Neal's Yard Remedies.
Mail Order: 0845 262 3145
Website: www.nealsyardremedies.com

Iredale Mineral Make-Up

Recommended by Sheherazade Goldsmith, editor of the 'green' book, *A Slice of Organic Life*, who uses these products on her sensitive skin. The range includes foundations, powders, lipsticks and glosses, eyeshadows, eyeliners and mascara.
Website: www.jiproducts.co.uk

Lily Lolo Mineral Cosmetics

Range includes foundations, powders, blushers, bronzers and eyeshadows. All products are parabens and fragrance free.
Website: www.lilylolo.co.uk

Medihoney Moisturising Cream

Contains various types of honey, including manuka, which have antibacterial and soothing, anti-inflammatory properties. Available from Victoria Health and pharmacies nationwide.
Telephone: 0800 3898 195
Website: www.victoriahealth.com

Oilatum

A range of products containing light liquid paraffin that leave a moisture-retaining film on the skin. For the treatment of dry skin conditions. Includes creams, soap, lotion, bath formula and scalp treatment.
Website: www.stiefel.co.uk

PetalCleanse

A surfactant-based lotion that removes allergens from the coats of cats and dogs. PetalCleanse has been independently tested and found to be safe for pets and effective in reducing symptoms in over 90 per cent of people allergic to pets.
Website: www.healthy-house.co.uk

ProbioStart

A probiotic supplement for pregnant and breastfeeding women, and infants six months and over. Research suggests that probiotics can lessen the risk of developing eczema.

Website: www.dtecta.co.uk

Salcura

A range of nutrient-based skincare products, developed to promote self-healing by bio-medical research scientist Dr Martin Schiele. Products include bath oil, shower gel and face and body hydrators – all of which are certified free from steroids, cortisones, alcohol, antibiotics, parabens and peroxides. Ingredients include vitamins, minerals, amino acids, essential oils and essential fatty acids.

Telephone: 01472 245 681
Email: info@salcura.com
Website: www.salcura.com

Showerhead with Vitamin C Filter

A shower filter that uses vitamin C to remove chlorine, a common skin irritant, from water.

Telephone: 08707 455 002
Website: www.allergybestbuys.co.uk

Skin Salveation

A range of skin products, shampoo and wash powder based on a soap originally devised by a group of Durham miners to help counteract dry and inflamed skin caused by their jobs. A local GP noted positive results among 200 patients. The products create a protective layer that allows the skin to heal.

Website: www.skinsalveation.com

The Soap Kitchen

Sells a range of ingredients from which you can make your own cleaning products, such as borax, bicarbonate of soda and essential oils. See also Chapter 4 – Home Front.

Address: Units 2 D&E Hatchmoor Industrial Estate, Hatchmoor Road, Torrington, Devon EX38 7HP

Telephone: 01805 622 944

Website: www.thesoapkitchen.co.uk

Surcare Sensitive Concentrated Washing-up Liquid

If you're prone to hand eczema, it's recommended that you wear protective gloves. If you're allergic to latex – or simply dislike wearing gloves for washing up – this product has been specially formulated to help prevent the irritation of sensitive skin. Surcare washing-up liquid is free from dye or perfume and it's concentrated, so only a small amount is needed. Other products in the Surcare range include automatic washing powder, laundry tablets, concentrated laundry liquid and fabric conditioner.

Website: www.surcare.co.uk

Therapeutic Skincare

A range of skin products which contain plant ingredients and essential oils and no harsh chemicals, especially designed for eczema sufferers. A shampoo is also available.

Website: www.gentlebodycare.co.uk

Uvistat Suncare

A brand of sun lotions and suncreams suitable for sensitive skin – traditionally prescribed by GPs and dermatologists. They all provide five star UVA protection as well as UVB protection – they're available in SPFs 20, 30 and 50. All products are water resistant for up to five hours and are hypo-allergenic.

Website: www.uvistat.com

Vinalac Probiotic Formula

A probiotic supplement for pregnant and breastfeeding women, produced by Novogen. It contains Lactobacillus rhamnosus; studies have suggested that it reduces the risk of children developing eczema. Website: www.probiotics4infanthealth.com

White Cotton Gloves

Soft, 100 per cent cotton gloves that allow children to play safely with glue, paints or animals, protecting damaged skin on hands, wrists or fingers. They're also ideal for adults to wear during the day under work gloves and useful at night after applying creams or emollients. Website: www.allergybestbuys.co.uk

Zambesia Botanica

A range of products, including a herbal moisturising cream containing extracts from the Kigelia Africana (sausage) tree. Africans have traditionally used this tree's bark, roots and fruit for its skincare properties – especially for dry, itchy skin conditions. Other products in the range include Scalp Application and Shampoo for dry, itchy, eczematous scalps and Moisturising Wash, which can be used in the bath or shower.
Website: www.all-ages-vitamins.co.uk

Helpful Books

Armstrong-Brown, Sue, *The Eczema Solution* (Vermillion, 2002) – outlines the six week habit-reversal programme, aimed at breaking the scratching habit, which is taught to patients at Chelsea and Westminster Hospital. It's claimed that positive results can be achieved within 21 days. The author has suffered from atopic eczema all of her life and over the years she tried every known 'cure' for her eczema, without success. After a referral to the Chelsea and Westminster Hospital she completed the Noren habit-reversal programme and she claims to have been free of eczema ever since.

Grossbart, Ted and Sherman, Carl, *Skin Deep: A Mind/Body Program for Healthy Skin* (Health Press, 1992) – this book explores the idea that skin is sensitive to emotions and suggests psychological techniques that may help to improve skin disorders. If you've tried conventional eczema treatments without success and you suspect stress or emotions trigger your eczema, this book is well worth a read.

Waterford, Kathleen, *The Skin Cure Diet: Heal Eczema from the Inside Out* (iUniverse, 2005) – this book is written by an eczema sufferer who believes that a yeast infection (candida) was responsible for her severe eczema. The aim of the book is to help people heal their eczema with a natural diet, rather than relying on drugs, creams, lotions or other medicines. If conventional treatments haven't helped you, Waterford's approach might. It's strongly recommended you take advice from your GP or a dietician before following any of the dietary changes suggested in the book. For more details go to her website: www.geocities.com/skincurediet.

Worth, Jennifer, *Eczema and Food Allergy – the Hidden Cause?* (Merton Books, 2007) – this book is written by a nursing sister who suffered from severe eczema apparently caused by food intolerances. Whilst her case was extreme, she suggests that some other people with eczema are suffering because of food intolerances. Worth reading if your eczema is severe and you've tried following a healthy diet and lifestyle and conventional treatments to no avail. It's strongly recommended you take advice from your GP or a dietician before following any of the dietary changes outlined in this book

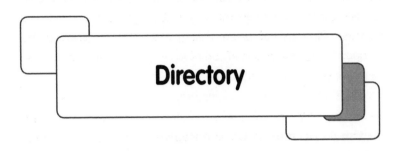

Directory

Below is a list of contacts which offer information and support for eczema sufferers.

ABC of Yoga
A website offering tips, advice and poses for those who wish to practise yoga at home. Also provides meditation techniques.
Website: www.abc-of-yoga.com

Allergy UK (Formerly The British Allergy Foundation)
National medical charity for people with allergies, food intolerances and chemical sensitivity. Provides up-to-date information on all aspects of allergy, as well as a nationwide network of support contacts who offer advice and support to fellow sufferers. Also runs three product endorsement schemes to help allergy sufferers select 'allergy friendly' products, as well as listing alerts on allergens in particular products.
Address: Allergy UK, 3 White Oak Square, London Road, Swanley, Kent, BR8 7AG Telephone: 01322 619 898
Email: info@allergyuk.org
Website: www.allergyuk.org

Blossom

A children's campaign from Allergy UK that aims to provide support to childhood allergy sufferers and their families.

Address: Blossom Campaign, Allergy UK, 3 White Oak Square, London Road, Swanley, Kent, BR8 7AG

Telephone: 01322 619 898

Website: www.blossomcampaign.org

British Association of Dermatologists

Provides a wide range of reliable information about the skin and skin diseases.

Telephone: 0207 383 0266

Website:www.bad.org.uk

The British Skin Foundation

A UK charity dedicated to skin disease (including eczema) research. Provides information about a range of skin conditions.

Website: www.britishskinfoundation.org.uk

British Society of Allergy and Clinical Immunology

Professional society of allergists and clinical immunologists. Lists specialist NHS Allergy Clinics in the UK.

Website: www.bsaci.org

British Wheel of Yoga

The national governing body for yoga in the UK, with a nationwide network of over 3,000 teachers.

Website: www.bwy.org.uk

Dermatology.co.uk

An independent website that provides an educational resource for skin conditions, including eczema, for the public, patients and health professionals.

Website: www.dermatology.co.uk

DermNet

Website of the New Zealand Dermatological Society Incorporated. Aims to present authoritative facts about the skin for patients and health professionals.

Website: www.dermnetnz.org

Eczemaletters

An American website offering easily understood information about eczema, written by dermatologists.

Website: www.eczemaletters.com

Eczema Mailing List

An automated mailing list which enables people with eczema to share their experiences with fellow sufferers.

Website: www.eczema.ndo.co.uk

EczemaNet

Website run by the American Academy of Dermatologists, offering up-to-date information on the treatment and management of eczema.

Website: www.skincarephysicians.com/eczemanet

The Eczema Society of Canada

Provides information about eczema and its treatment, as well as encouraging and funding research and increasing public awareness of the condition. The website is run by parents of young eczema sufferers who receive treatment at the Hospital for Sick Children, Toronto, Canada, and doctors who practise in the dermatology department.

Address: Eczema Society of Canada, 417 The Queensway South, PO Box 25009, Keswick, Ontario, L4P 2C4

Telephone: 00 1 905 535 0776

Website: www.eczemahelp.ca

Eczema Voice

A friendly eczema forum with lots of related features and services.

Address: Eczema Voice, PO Box 5448, Milton Keynes, MK4 1XJ

Website: www.eczemavoice.com

Foods Matter

Offers information on food allergies and intolerances.

Address : Foods Matter, 5 Lawn Road, London NW3 2XS

Telephone: 020 7722 2866

E-mail: info@foodsmatter.com

Website: www.foodsmatter.com

The Henry Spink Foundation

An independent charity created to help families of children with severe disabilities of all kinds. Provides information on conventional and alternative medicine, therapies and research relating to a wide range of physical and mental disorders. Includes a large section on candida, which some people believe is implicated in some cases of eczema.

Address: c/o Montgomery Swann, Scotts Sufferance Wharf, 1 Mill Street, London, SE1 2DE

Website: www.henryspink.org

National Eczema Society

Organisation dedicated to the needs of people with eczema, dermatitis and sensitive skin. Offers practical information and support to people with eczema, their carers and health professionals wanting to learn more about the condition.

Address: Hill House, Highgate Hill, London, N19 5NA
Helpline: 0800 089 1122
Telephone: 0207 281 3553
Website: www.eczema.org

The Royal College of Pathologists

Offers information to allergy sufferers and their relatives.
Telephone: 0207 451 6733
Email: webmaster@rcpath.org
Website: www.rcpath.org

Royal London Homoeopathic Hospital

The hospital's Allergy, Environmental & Nutritional Medicine Clinic specialises in the diagnosis and treatment of patients with allergic and other conditions in which diet or environmental factors may play a part.

Address: Allergy, Environmental & Nutritional Medicine Clinic, Great Ormond Street, London, WC1N 3HR
Telephone: 020 7391 8888

The Skin Care Campaign

Campaigns nationally to the government and the NHS on behalf of skin patients.
Website: www.skincarecampaign.org

Skin Care World

A website run by Molnlycke Healthcare, who manufacture Epaderm. The site offers resources, information and a message board for people suffering from eczema and other skin problems such as psoriasis. Includes advice from Dr Chris Steele – the resident doctor on ITV's *This Morning* programme.

Website: www.skincareworld.co.uk

TalkEczema

An eczema support website set up by Deborah Mason, an eczema sufferer, as a result of her young daughter's severe atopic eczema. It's a useful site offering information about eczema, an A–Z of treatments, a newsletter, chat room, features and personal stories.

Website: www.talkeczema.com

Transcendal Meditation

Offers information about the benefits of transcendental meditation and a list of qualified teachers

Website: www.t-m.org.uk

Under My Skin

A website offering up-to-date information about eczema.

Website: www.undermyskin.co.uk

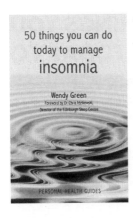

50 THINGS YOU CAN DO TODAY TO MANAGE INSOMNIA

Wendy Green

ISBN: 978 84024 723 7

Paperback   £4.99

Do you lie awake in bed worrying about things
you have to do the next day?

Do you get up feeling tired and as if
you haven't had enough sleep?

If so, you could be suffering from insomnia. In this easy-to-follow book, Wendy Green explains the sleep/wake cycle, and offers practical advice and a holistic approach to help you combat insomnia, including simple lifestyle and dietary changes and DIY complementary therapies.

'... this book helpfully provides a comprehensive rundown of everything that might impact on sleep and help the insomniac... All in all a fun read in which even the most committed insomniac will find solace'

Dr Chris Idzikowski, director of the Edinburgh Sleep Centre

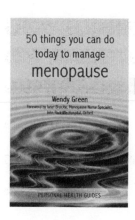

50 things you can do
today to manage
menopause

Wendy Green
Foreword by Janet Brockie, Menopause Nurse Specialist,
John Radcliffe Hospital, Oxford

PERSONAL HEALTH GUIDES

50 THINGS YOU CAN DO TODAY TO MANAGE MENOPAUSE

Wendy Green

ISBN: 978 84024 720 6

Paperback   £4.99

Do you think you might be going through the menopause?

Are you confused by conflicting advice about HRT?

In this easy-to-follow book, Wendy Green explains the common physical and psychological symptoms of menopause and offers practical advice and a holistic approach to help you deal with them, including simple lifestyle and dietary changes and DIY complementary therapies.

'*This book, with its friendly, easy-going style, offers a wide breadth of information and valuable practical advice to meet all needs. It embraces the diversity of women's experiences and responds to their differences*'

Janet Brockie, menopause nurse specialist,
John Radcliffe Hospital, Oxford

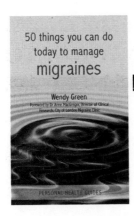

50 THINGS YOU CAN DO TODAY TO MANAGE MIGRAINES

Wendy Green

ISBN: 978 84024 722 0

Paperback   £4.99

Do you suffer from severe headaches, sometimes with nausea and visual impairment?

Can these headaches last for up to a day or longer at a time?

If so, you could be experiencing migraines. In this easy-to-follow book, Wendy Green explains how dietary, psychological and environmental factors can cause migraines, and offers practical advice and a holistic approach to help you manage them, including simple lifestyle and dietary changes and DIY complementary therapies.

'Wendy Green outlines the variety of treatments that are available over the counter, and also gives an overview of what is available from a GP… It may not yet be possible to 'cure' migraines but it is possible to lead a normal life despite them'

Dr Anne MacGregor, director of clinical research,
City of London Migraine Clinic

www.summersdale.com

Have you enjoyed this book?
If so, why not write a review on your favourite website?
Thanks very much for buying this Summersdale book.